D0685567

Ultimate Training

Ultimate Training

Gary Null's Complete Guide
to Eating Right, Exercising,
and Living Longer

▼

Gary Null and
Dr. Howard Robins

St. Martin's Press   New York

DESIGN BY JUDITH A. STAGNITTO

Library of Congress Cataloging-in-Publication Data

Null, Gary.
    Ultimate training : Gary Null's complete guide to eating right, exercising and living longer / Gary Null.
        p. cm.
    ISBN 0-312-08796-9 (pbk.)
    1. Runners (Sports)—Health and hygiene. 2. Runners (Sports)—Nutrition. 3. Running—Accidents and injuries—Prevention.
    I. Title.
    RC1220.R8N85 1993
    613.7'172—dc20   92-44033
                                                                           CIP

First Edition: April 1993

10 9 8 7 6 5 4 3 2 1

Contents

▼

Preface

▼

What?! Another book on walking and running? Haven't we seen a glut of those in the last five years?

Yes, but what holds true for all other subjects also is true of running: The potential for broadening our base of understanding always exists. I have read most books on running, power walking, nutrition, and exercise. Many are so scientific that they are of little use to the general reader; others are so general that they are of no use to the more advanced athlete. Some have emphasized technique, warm-up, or pre- and post-sports training; others have stressed the role of nutrition in exercise programs.

For the past twenty-five years, I have run competitively, participated in most sports, and actively studied and taught nutrition and health sciences. During that time, I have learned that we only begin to realize our full potential in any field of endeavor when we take a holistic approach that encompasses our physical, mental, and spiritual dimensions. This book presents such an approach to power walking and running, one based on the belief that all three dimensions are interdependent and indispensable in an exercise program.

Typically, a runner's diary includes space for the number of miles logged, blood pressure ratings, weight, and comments. This one, on the other hand, emphasizes attitude. What did you see when you looked in the mirror this morning? Who did you see? The answer to that question is essential. If your exercise program is designed to train the wrong person for the wrong reasons, then it's not going to have much real meaning for you.

This book is directed to the seekers of wholeness, wellness, and balance. In another society, in another place and time, these people may have found what they were looking for through Zen, meditation, and yoga. For many who live here and now, marathon training, exercising, and nutrition are the vehicles for this journey to well-being. That is my reason for contributing one more book to the many that exist on running.

Introduction: A True Fable

▼

by Gary Null

"Real life is doing something you love to do with your whole being."

—KRISHNAMURTI

Some time ago, a close friend of mine decided to start running. This man, an attorney, had lived his life in an average way and avoided all forms of exercise for many years. I learned of his newfound interest in health when he called me on the phone one morning and said, "I want to get ready for the marathon." Just like that. I asked him why.

He explained that in previous years, it had been relatively easy for him to attract people into his life. He was young, attractive, and financially secure—a successful lawyer with an important social position. But in the 1970s, he realized that his career was no longer enough to guarantee his popularity. He was also expected to have a beautiful body and to become involved in running or another physical discipline. And so, to keep up with the times, he decided to change his image by becoming a marathon runner. This, he hoped, would increase his value in the eyes of others and boost his self-esteem.

With that goal in mind, he directed all of his effort to running. Indeed, he pursued the sport with such passion, dedication, and discipline that he was able to complete his first marathon within one year. In four subsequent marathons, he improved his time with each race, achieving a "personal best" of 3:01. This success brought him the one major benefit that he desired, greater social acceptance.

Before long, however, his success began to fade away just as quickly as it had appeared. You see, my friend was more concerned with getting quick results than with the process of sustaining success. As a result, he overtrained. By the sixth marathon, he could no longer improve his time; by the seventh, he was actually losing ground, running slower than in any of his previous races.

With no more "personal bests" in sight, he lost his passion for running and quit the sport out of frustration. Over the next three years, he reverted to his old life-style except for an occasional jog in the park. He said that there was no point to the effort of running if he could not improve his time. He did not want to participate in anything that did not enhance his self-esteem. But he still found it socially advantageous to call himself a marathon runner. Although he had given up the actual sport, he continued to speak the jogger's language. He knew the terminology well and would use it to impress others.

In the 1980s, some new trends in the health field caught my friend's interest. With the same diligence formerly applied to running, he obtained books on all of the latest buzzwords—vegetarianism, new age, holism, transformation processing. Again, however, he was not motivated to comprehend these principles in a larger context. He had no real appreciation of vegetarianism and the health benefits that it offered. Unlike other vegetarians, his change in diet did not make a political statement meant to support organic farmers or a spiritual one to express reverence for all life. He wished only to grasp the idea and learn the basic jargon so that he could posture a more convincing image.

On the surface, he appeared to possess many sought-after qualities: He was educated, self-assured, aggressive, and financially independent. Many people envied him, but they did not see the loneliness and emptiness that he felt inside. He was always on the go, always looking to outer circumstances for fulfillment. Running was his stimulation for the 70s; diet and new-age disciplines his modi operandi for the 80s.

In retrospect, my friend knows that he chose to run for the wrong reasons. He was using the sport to improve his social status rather than to achieve real physical gains. He overtrained, ran himself into a state of exhaustion, and became prone to injury. The psychological benefits were minimal as well because his actions fed only the ego and not the true self. It was as if he were pouring attention, time, and money into a cardboard self; any discipline that would enhance his sense of self-esteem would do. Decades later, the result of all this misspent energy was a lack of spiritual direction.

My friend's experience teaches us all that we must explore the true motives behind our own actions. Many of us are not in touch with the highest part of our nature. Without an integrated system of beliefs, our lives may become a neurotic struggle. We forget that we do not have to prove anything to anyone, least of all ourselves, to be accepted as an individual.

Many athletes approach running and walking from a limited and false perspective. Some see it as an intellectual process in which they must meet specific goals, such as running one mile in five minutes. But when intellect alone controls an exercise program, the motivation to accomplish long-term goals will be lacking. Other athletes may operate from an emotional base, compulsively seeking to achieve "more" through running— more speed, more stamina, more strength. The desire for "more" may help them to avoid parts of themselves that they perceive to be "less" worthy. In that way, running can become a method of denying the self and covering up pain, much like going to a doctor for Valium.

The problems behind these failed approaches need not be viewed as irreversible, however. We can re-empower ourselves by accepting our fears and insecurities and working through them. We can choose to stop seeing our problems as insurmountable and start seeing them as opportunities for renewal and growth. We can use the conflicts that arise from a non-integrated belief system as points of transition. We can reinvest our energy in nourishing our true self rather than allow ourselves to be manipulated by a superficial ego.

Running, for the dedicated athlete, can be an integral part of this transformation process. When we train properly and holistically, we gain internal rewards rather than ones based on other people's expectations of us. We begin to tune in to the positive and negative aspects of ourselves and experience a full spectrum of feelings, from exhilaration to humility. The humility will come when we let go of our ego-dominated self, accept our limitations, and better understand that it is all right not to be perfect. Only then can we experience greater trust in all aspects of our lives and make way for real change to occur. Ultimately, this process will allow us to live in a more positive way.

Now that you are embarking on a new exercise program, I hope that you will approach it holistically, not simply as an extension of your ego needs and insecurities as my friend did. A true approach to athletics is meant to nourish the soul and the psyche, not merely the body. Consider what Krishnamurti, the profound Indian spiritual teacher, said: "Real life is doing something you love to do with your whole being." There should be no inner contradiction between what you are doing and what you want to be doing.

When this state is achieved, training becomes an integrated process that leads to tremendous joy. Your exercise program will not become boring, and you won't have to overcome the perennial inner debates—"I don't feel like running today, but I guess I really should . . ."—just to become motivated. Instead, the motivation to train will come from an inner feeling of being connected to the activity itself. When your health-promoting activities complement all other aspects of your life, you will honestly enjoy getting out of bed early in the morning to run. You will not resent the sweat that it produces or the time that it takes because fundamentally you will have become *all* of it.

Part One

Holistic Living

Chapter 1

▼

What Is Holism?

"Holism" reflects a balance of the natural forces around you and within you. To live your life in a holistic way, you must take the time each day to nourish the various elements of your being—the body, the mind, the spirit, and the life force that connects you to every living thing. In doing so, you will avoid the extremes that exhaust your life force. And the energy that you absorb and project will be a positive one.

Many people misunderstand the quest for "wholeness." The word itself implies that a person must acquire new knowledge to become whole. But the ability to do so is a natural part of your makeup that goes beyond the conscious level of awareness. Consider the body itself, for example. Even though you may be processing harmful foods and negative thoughts, your body is working hard to sustain a state of homeostasis. Trillions of cells function in perfect harmony to maintain your health.

It is an exciting theory that speculates that these living cells are guided by a higher consciousness as they work together in magnificent unison. The balance within your own body is a microcosm of the harmony inherent in the larger universe. As you begin to recognize your intrinsically perfect nature, you will be drawn to the thoughts and actions that help you to eliminate destructive tendencies and further rebalance your life.

Where does the quest for balance begin? Start by taking an inventory of yourself that helps you to understand exactly who you are. This means coming to grips with your true self, not the superficial package of achievements and mannerisms that we present to the world each day. The point is to conduct an honest evaluation of yourself without looking to others for answers. Although a good teacher can help you tune in to yourself without projecting his or her own values and expectations, most people's perceptions of your needs will be colored by their own feelings and beliefs. Others can guide you on your journey, but you alone hold the key to becoming more balanced.

You can alleviate much of the tension and anxiety that you feel—and allow your potential to unfold naturally—by trusting yourself and recognizing that you already have control of your life. As you become more centered, you'll spend less time trying to "figure out" life. Your questions will be answered intuitively, and you will be able to approach life in a more productive and creative way. You'll also get more out of each day as you reprioritize your schedule to allow time to eat properly, train fully, relax, meditate, socialize, and work in a balanced and unhurried manner. From this perspective, even distressing problems can become a channel to growth. Disease can be viewed as nature's way of saying that you are out of balance and that you need to confront, embrace, and transcend certain important conflicts in your life.

The athlete who negates holism and forces his discipline also will negate the self and feed his insecurities. And the more insecure a person feels, the harder the effort will be. After a while, this athlete may find it impossible to surpass new goals. He may become depressed and anxious as he focuses on self-styled limitations rather than on the limitless possibilities.

By contrast, a holistic perspective will make running, walking, or any athletic endeavor a joyful experience. The athlete can surrender to the process of the sport and overcome the need to achieve specific goals. The sport then becomes a paradigm for achieving balance in other areas of your life. It reflects the degree of self-love that you have.

When it comes to training, attitude is everything. If you run with a competitive mind and believe that you have to "win," you will limit the very process of growth. But if you forget about external rewards and run for your total health instead, then it will not matter how fast you go, whether or not you win, and what your image is in the eyes of others.

4

▼

Part Two

The Holistic Approach to Running

Chapter 2

▼

Benefits of Running

Running's beneficial effects on the body have been proven quite convincingly over the years. The heart, circulation, immune apparatus, musculoskeletal system, and ability to handle stress all improve from a power-walking and running program. Although runners can get circulatory problems, heart disorders, and cancer just like everyone else, of course, running often prevents these problems or reduces their severity. It also bolsters the autoimmune system and helps to remove toxins from the body.

The circulatory and cardiovascular systems, in particular, benefit from running. A regular program can reduce your heart rate and increase stroke volume. The heart can then supply more blood with each stroke, thereby meeting the body's needs with fewer strokes. Improved circulation affects the body in several ways. First, it regulates the blood pressure and prevents fatty acids from depositing in the arteries. It also enhances the supply of oxygen to the brain and the removal of waste products, which prevents or lessens senility and the hardening of arteries. The size and strength of the blood vessels and arteries increases, as does the number of capillaries. This allows more blood to flow to the organs and tissues, thereby halting the death of cells and prolonging life.

Running also enhances the musculoskeletal system by strengthening muscles throughout the entire body. Osteoporosis, or the depletion of calcium in the bones, may be prevented by a running program as well. From the age of about thirty-five until they reach menopause, women can lose up to 2 percent of their calcium per year. After that, the loss can run as high as 5 percent each year. Men, by contrast, lose about 1 percent per year after the age of sixty. This condition may be avoided through running, which causes calcium to be reabsorbed in the bones through gravitational pressure. The force created by the pull of muscles on bones also facilitates the reabsorption process.

Finally, running is an effective stress reducer. The relaxation that results from running can increase circulation to the brain and lower your blood pressure. It also reduces muscle tension and helps to prevent the problems that a tense body can create, including muscle injuries, decreased energy, and headaches. Studies show that runners are better equipped to handle psychological problems and that they tend to suffer less from depression. Not surprisingly, long-distance runners also excel in business. Your work can only benefit when you feel less stress, maintain high energy levels, and enhance your self-image, all of which can be gained from running and power walking.

Chapter 3
▼

Running and Your Heart Rate

In designing a running program, you must determine the optimum heart-rate levels that you want to reach during the exercise period. The American College of Sports Medicine recommends that aerobic exercises such as running be performed three to five days per week. During a 15- to 60-minute exercise period, a healthy person's heart rate (the number of beats per minute) should equal 60 to 90 percent of his or her *maximum* rate.

Each person's maximum heart rate depends on his or her

age. To determine this rate, simply subtract your age from the number 220. The result is the most number of times that your heart should ever beat per minute. Highly conditioned athletes may add another 10 percent. For the purposes of running and other aerobic workouts, however, you must establish a 60 to 90 percent "target range" of this maximum rate—and then stay within that range. Anything less than 60 percent will not tax the heart enough to produce results; anything in excess of 90 percent could prove too strenuous.

A healthy forty-year-old, for example, would calculate his or her maximum rate and target range as follows:

$$\textit{Maximum rate:}$$
$$220 - 40 = 180$$

$$\textit{Low target:}$$
$$60\% \text{ of } 180 = \frac{180 \times 60}{100}$$
$$= 108$$

$$\textit{High target:}$$
$$90\% \text{ of } 180 = \frac{180 \times 90}{100}$$
$$= 162$$

During the course of running, use your pulse count to determine whether your heart rate is within the target range. Your wrist or temple will provide the most accurate pulse reading. Do not use the carotid artery in your neck because the rate may slow down when you press on this artery. If your pulse rate is a bit high during the exercise period, either run slower or use less vigorous motions to lessen your energy output; if your pulse is too low, run a little harder to increase it.

Through regular exercise, you will decrease your resting rate because the heart begins to operate more efficiently, pumping more blood with fewer strokes. The average resting pulse rate for men is 80; for women, 72. For those in good condition, the resting rate often is much lower. As your conditioning improves and your resting rate lowers, you will have to run harder to reach the target range. After running, the amount of time that it takes your heart to return to its resting rate provides a good indication of fitness. Take your pulse as soon as you stop and every few minutes after that. Then judge your recovery rate according to these guidelines: 6 to 8 minutes indicates good condition; 8 to 10 minutes indicates fair condition; more than 10 minutes indicates poor condition. Eventually, it should take less time to recover, providing you with measurable evidence of fitness improvements.

With any type of aerobic work, the cardiovascular benefits are greatest during the first 20 to 30 minutes of exercise. Beyond that, you still benefit but to a lesser degree. Therefore, the best approach is to maintain a regular schedule that gets your heart rate into the target area for 30 minutes at least three times a week. Keep in mind that skipping a few days of running won't disrupt the program, but skipping a couple of weeks will.

To determine how energetically you should run on any given day, take your pulse before you get out of bed in the morning and compare it to your average awakening rate. (This can be determined by taking your pulse immediately upon awakening each morning for a week and then dividing the total by seven.) Ease up on your exercise if the rate is two to three beats faster per minute that day; avoid aerobic exercise entirely if the rate is five to six beats faster. When the rate exceeds the norm by that amount, it means the body is already stressed. The warm-up and stretching exercises contained in this book can help you balance your systems and reduce stress on those particular days.

Chapter 4

▼

Injury-Free Running

At one time or another, almost everyone who exercises will experience a minor injury of some sort, such as sore muscles. But in most cases, an effective injury-prevention program can help to reduce the incidence of severe or chronic injuries. In *The Physician and Sports Medicine* (McGraw-Hill, 1984), cardiologist George Sheehan, M.D., maintained that certain structural weaknesses in his body led to most of his minor injuries, for example. Running style, the condition of the terrain, and the type of running shoes used all contributed to the anatomical imperfections and caused injuries. In addition, an improper approach to warming up, stretching, and cooling down would affect his running regimen. By recognizing and correcting these problems, Dr. Sheehan ran with relatively few injuries for years.

It's always better to prevent an injury than to treat one after the fact. However, sore or achy muscles when you begin a new exercise program or revive an old one must be expected. The guidelines presented here will help you to reduce the incidence of injury or recover more quickly if you do experience a problem:

1. Build up your running pace slowly. Speed will develop naturally with time and practice. Do not do too much, too fast, too soon.

2. Warm up properly each time you run.

3. Pay attention to proper form and technique. An exercise done incorrectly can harm your body.

4. Take note of your environment. Watch out for everything from potholes to pollution levels when you are running.

5. Stretch and cool down properly after exercising.

6. Allow plenty of time to complete the entire exercise program without rushing.

7. Drink plenty of water before, during, and after exercising.

8. When beginning a new sport or exercise program, get good instruction and then have your form and technique checked from time to time.

9. Exercise at a comfortable level or until strong discomfort begins. Do *not* continue past this discomfort to the point of pain.

10. If you become injured, don't quit exercising altogether. Instead, choose another form of exercise that you can safely perform. In the event of a serious injury, of course, you must first treat the injury and then decide what type of exercise will promote healing.

11. Never try to diagnose yourself when you suffer a serious injury or experience a lot of pain. Many running injuries have similar symptoms and more serious problems may develop later on if you do not properly identify the nature of the injury. A doctor can diagnose the true source of the problem and may recommend an appropriate therapy. The final choice, of course, is yours.

12. Scale back on exercising if your heartbeat is two to three times higher than your usual resting rate. If it is five to six beats higher, do all of the pre-run and post-run exercises covered in Chapter 18. But do not run or perform other types of strenuous aerobic or anaerobic work that will put more stress on the body.

13. Wear clothing that accommodates both the type of exercise to be performed and the weather.

14. Use only high-quality equipment in your workouts, whether it be running shoes, tennis rackets, or exercise bikes. Supplies of a poor grade will diminish performance and increase the risk of injury. Shop carefully for good-

quality (though not necessarily expensive) equipment. Consumer reports and other athletes can guide you to the best sources. Once you purchase the equipment, be sure to maintain and repair it when necessary.

15. Work some flexibility into your exercise program to avoid a rigid routine. Studies indicate that overexercising or an anxious workout can do more harm than good. To avoid compulsive, goal-oriented exercising, incorporate a range of activities and energy levels into your program. When the program is unchanging, you may go through the motions so routinely that you do not really experience and benefit from the workout.

A final note on injury prevention: Running is a sport that involves your entire body, not just your feet and legs. All of your internal systems interact with one another when you run. These include the musculoskeletal, circulatory, respiratory, genito-urinary, gastrointestinal, and endocrine systems. By recognizing that running affects all of these functions, you can better appreciate the effect that exercise has on your body and learn to prevent injuries.

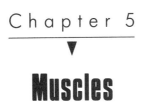

Chapter 5
▼
Muscles

To prevent muscle injuries, which affect runners quite often, it helps to understand some basic concepts about muscle functioning. First, the composition: According to William K. McArdle, a prominent exercise physiologist, muscles contain 75 percent water, 20 percent protein, and 5 percent other ingredients, including inorganic salts, enzymes, fats, carbohydrates, and pigments. During demanding workouts, such as long-distance running, says McArdle, the muscles consume about seventy times more oxygen than when they are resting.

The muscles are composed of two types of fibers: fast-twitch and slow-twitch. The fast-twitch variety provides rapid power and energy from an anaerobic system, such as a lack of oxygen when one is sprinting. The slow-twitch fibers function better in an aerobic state that supplies more oxygen to the body, such as during long-distance running. Hence, successful runners with great endurance have more slow-twitch muscle fibers.

In addition, exercise physiologists have identified a third type of muscle fiber, called Class 1B, which can assume either fast- or slow-twitch properties. Long-distance runners, for example, can enhance their performance in two ways—by developing their natural slow-twitch fibers and by changing any fast-twitch Class 1B fibers into slow-twitch fibers. This process will take quite some time, but it can be achieved through long-term and persistent training.

Running will increase the size of your muscle fibers, thereby enlarging the muscles themselves. Running removes fat from the muscles and makes them more compact. As the fat burns off and larger muscle masses develop, your body may become leaner even if you do not lose actual weight. While men can develop larger muscle masses because they have higher testosterone levels, women can run as well as most men and surpass them in training and racing.

To strengthen muscles, you must overload them by increasing the amount of stress you place on the fibers. That's why an unvarying running schedule—with identical distances, levels of stress, and pacing every day—will not challenge the body. Keep trying to improve until you've reached a peak level of running; in doing so, you will also achieve your maximum level of overall health and fitness.

Clearly, running has a tremendous impact on muscles. That's why a variety of injuries, from strains and cramps to shin splints and hamstring pulls, can occur. What follows is a discussion of the common muscle injuries and related therapies.

Strains

A muscle can become strained in any of three places, including where it starts (the weakest part), in the main belly, and where it inserts into the bone. Muscle injuries, which occur frequently in runners, fall into the same classes as tendinitis I, II, and III. With a Class I strain, the muscle fibers are stretched beyond their usual limits. This may occur when you run too hard, too fast, or too far without first warming up the muscles. Class II strains show a partial tearing of fibers, while Class III strains signify a complete tearing of the muscle.

The first two classes of muscle strain occur most often; Class III strains rarely stem from running. A muscle strain can be treated with elevation of the affected area and massage. The other muscles and tissues that surround the strained area also must be stretched and strengthened.

Cramps

A number of factors can contribute to muscle cramping, including dehydration during exercise, overuse of muscles, mineral deficiencies, and stretch reflex contractions. The latter type of spasm usually occurs at night when you are sleeping. You can alleviate reflex contractions by stretching before you go to bed. Be sure to warm up first by lying on your back and "bicycling" gently with your legs in the air for 1 to 2 minutes.

Dehydration may cause cramps during a workout, often following one or more hours of exercise. Drink plenty of water as a preventative measure. Chronic cramps, on the other hand, may signal a salt deficiency. See a doctor if you have this condition and eat more foods that contain natural salt. Cramps that occur in various muscles at different times may indicate a lack of such minerals as calcium, magnesium, and potassium. Again, eat more foods that are rich with these minerals.

Cramps from the overuse of muscles may result when you do "too much, too fast, too soon," the surest route to injury. A new athlete or one who is out of practice may develop these cramps by increasing the level of activity too quickly. The best advise is to take it slow, allowing your muscles to strengthen gradually.

DOMS

Delayed Onset Muscle Soreness (DOMS) may occur soon after you begin a program of strenuous exercise. The demands placed on the muscles cause them to become inflamed, creating pain and stiffness anywhere from one to four days after the workout has ended. The soreness may last from thirty minutes to several days. The athletes most susceptible to DOMS are those who work out intermittently (such as on weekends), those who are beginners to a sport, and those who return to an activity too quickly.

You can help prevent DOMS by using fluid movements, rather than choppy ones, during your workout. In addition, focus on staying flexible with a comprehensive warm-up and cool-down routine. If DOMS does occur, most experts recommend a "hair of the dog treatment." That is, treat the exercised-induced soreness with more exercise. It really helps!

Shin Splints

Long-distance running may lead to two different types of shin splints, both of which create pain in the lower leg. The first type, an anterior compartment shin split, occurs in the front of the leg when running puts a heavy strain on several muscles of the shin. These muscles pull away from the bone and cause swelling. A "compartment" is created between the muscle and bone, trapping lymph fluid from the body tissues. The hydrostatic pressure (from the fluid) then presses on the nerves and causes pain.

The resulting pain or tightness may occur during or after running. Oftentimes, the pain can be alleviated by elevating and icing the affected area. You may want to wrap the lower leg with an elastic bandage as well. A better approach, of course, is to prevent the shin splint from happening in the first place. In most cases, anterior compartment splints are caused by tightness in the rear leg muscles. Stretching after running can loosen the muscles and prevent the injury.

In some cases, these shin splints occur when you take exceptionally long strides while running. Shorten your strides if this appears to be the case. Other ways to prevent shin splints include running on a softer surface and using heel cushions. Orthotic devices also will help those people with a structural foot imbalance, especially when used in conjunction with other preventative measures.

Posterior compartment shin splints, the second type, occur deeper behind the muscles in front of the lower leg. They, too, involve more than one muscle. In most cases, however, they are caused by an imbalance of the foot called overpronation, or the "hypermobile foot," which is the inward twisting of the ankle and a flattening of the arch.

Orthotic devices similar to arch supports can prevent posterior compartment splints by controlling hypermobility. And again, the rear leg muscles must be properly stretched. The time-honored RICE (rest, ice, compression, and elevation) treatment also should lessen the pain. A great way to ice the shins is to fill a Styrofoam cup with water and freeze it. Use the cup to ice the shins in a circular motion, moving from the ankle to the knee. Peel away the cup as the ice melts.

Plantar Fasciitis

When the muscle beneath the arch of the foot becomes strained, this musculotendonous injury will occur. The muscle in question stretches from the front of the heel bone to the ball of the foot, or metatarsals. The soreness or pain usually begins after running, when you wake up in the morning, or following a long period of inactivity. The first few steps are accompanied by a tightness or soreness, which eventually starts to dissipate.

A hypermobile foot causes the overstretching of this muscle. Plantar fasciitis also creates trigger points in the calf; these points are small spots of muscle that have died over energy areas. In this case, such procedures as acupressure, acupuncture, and shiatsu will relieve the pain. RICE and massage can also provide relief. Do not use cortisone injections, however, for the treatment of such injuries. The cortisone will weaken tissues.

As with preventing shin splints, the rear leg muscles must be stretched to avoid plantar fasciitis. When the rear leg muscles are tight, they cause the muscles on the bottom of the foot to contract, leading to plantar fascia strains. This relationship illustrates how the body parts interrelate: By stretching the rear leg muscles, you can help the foot; by running with your feet in the proper position, you can help the rear leg muscles.

A running shoe that is too short for your foot can also cause this condition. When you walk or run, your foot moves forward ⅛ to ¾ inch, regardless of how tightly you tie your shoes. Therefore, short shoes will eventually cause a tightening of the plantar fascia muscles and possibly lead to an injury. To avoid this problem, allow some extra length in your shoes, typically about one inch or a "thumbnail" from the tip of your longest toe to the end of the shoe.

Hamstring Injury

Runners often suffer from an injury to the hamstrings, the muscles that stretch between the buttocks and the upper half of the lower legs. The typical symptoms—spasms, soreness, pain, and swelling—can occur anywhere between the hip and the foot. Most often, however, the pain concentrates in the middle or upper part of the back of the leg. If you experience pain when you try to straighten your leg at the knee, it's a good indication that you have a hamstring injury.

The primary causes of hamstring injuries are stretching too much before you run and too little afterward. As you run, the hamstrings become tighter and stronger; when you finish, they may tighten up even more. Therefore, you must do a lot of post-workout stretching to loosen and relax the muscles. The stretches described in Chapter 18 will do the job.

An imbalance in the pelvis may cause hamstring injuries by chronically tightening the muscles. A chiropractor or osteopath can correct this problem by realigning the pelvis and back bones. In other instances, structural imbalances of the foot may contribute to hamstring problems. In that case, a podiatrist can control the condition with orthotics. Keep in mind that all injuries must be accurately diagnosed as soon as possible. The nature of the injury and all possible causes must be identified. Once that has been done, you and your doctor can choose an appropriate therapy.

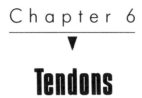

Chapter 6

▼

Tendons

Tendons, which connect muscles to bones, are thick, fibrous bands at the end of a muscle. When the lining of a tendon becomes inflamed, or if a tendon is strained to its limit or torn, a condition called tendinitis occurs. Most often, tendinitis will affect three areas of the feet and legs: the Achilles tendon, located just above the heel; the quadriceps, which are the four greater extensor muscles in the front of the thigh; and the perineal and extensor tendons, which run between the middle of the lower leg and the foot.

Class I tendinitis occurs when the fibers are stretched beyond their tolerable limits. If swelling and soreness result, alleviate these problems by resting the affected area. With a Class II injury, the fibers are partially torn. The swelling and pain will be much greater than with Class I tendinitis. Again, 24 to 48 hours of rest will facilitate the healing process. A Class III injury means that the fibers are completely torn.

When a tendon is injured, the first course of action is to stop the initial swelling. The following massage should do the job: Rub the injured area with short, fast, gentle strokes in the direction of your stomach. This causes the fluids to drain toward the body's major fluid collection points, our lymphnodes. Continue for 30 seconds, stroking in one direction only. Switch to firm, slow strokes in the same direction. If you still feel pain, go back to the short, fast strokes for another 30 seconds. Repeat the process until the pain has stopped or greatly lessened. This method can be used during the first 24 to 48 hours, along with rest, elevation, and ice.

With more severe tendinitis, apply ice immediately to control the swelling. It should take about 10 minutes of ice massage, rubbing in a counterclockwise motion, to numb the affected area. Following a few minutes of pain, the area will start to tingle and then become numb. Applying transverse friction with the ice will reduce the inflammation as well. Via this method, you rub quickly and firmly across the tendon, as if playing a violin. If the area is too tender, simply place a bag of ice on the tendon for 20 minutes. With an acute injury, in particular, this method can help reduce the swelling and pain. You can elevate the affected area and compress it with an elastic bandage as well.

A combination of heat and massage can alleviate minor pains, stiffness, and swelling. One quick and easy method is to place a hot towel on the injured tendon, changing the towel every ten to fifteen minutes. This simple technique can produce the same results as hydroculator packs and other expensive methods of heat application. Whirlpools and hot baths can also be effective, especially when combined with a massage. The massage will stretch the fibers back to their normal length and break up the spasms and scar tissues that cause pain and limit motion. With mild cases of tendinitis, the pain should subside in two to three days. If it does not, or if you experience extreme pain immediately following the injury, consult a physician.

The next step is to alternate passive and active stretching to recondition the injured tendon. Passive and gentle exercises will warm up the tendon. The more powerful, active exercises will help stretch the tightened tendon back to its pre-injury length. Remember to strengthen the muscles surrounding the injured tendon. They will somewhat relieve the pressure on the tendon and allow you to return more quickly to running.

Use the "functional progressions" described in Chapter 8 when you return to running. Be aware that any tendon injury will change your running form. If you ignore the injury, you will begin to compensate and create problems in other parts of your body. Since a compensation problem is harder to correct than the original injury, you should run until you feel strong discomfort, but not beyond that point. Pay attention to what your body is telling you and don't use medicine to disguise any discomfort.

An inflammation of the Achilles tendon, which is caused by tight rear leg muscles, merits special consideration. Treat Achilles tendinitis immediately with RICE, followed by stretching and strengthening exercises. Orthotic devices for your feet can also help to prevent and treat this injury. The devices position your feet properly for running. If you use heel lifts, be sure to put them in *both* shoes to maintain your body's balance.

An exception to this rule, of course, is a case where one leg is functionally shorter than the other due to a non-aligned pelvis. Unequal leg length can cause a tightening of the Achilles tendon in either leg or both, making a person more prone to tendinitis. Try to correct the problem at its source by having the back and pelvis professionally realigned. If necessary, a heel lift can be used to compensate for the exact difference in length with a true, structurally shorter leg.

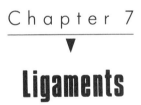

Chapter 7
▼
Ligaments

Ligaments are small bands of strong and flexible tissue that stabilize your joints. They connect from one bone to another, holding the joints in place. The ligaments can be sprained or torn, resulting in Class I, II, or III injuries, when they become short and tight due to inadequate training and improper body positioning during running. Poor body positioning is a structural bone problem that may be inherited or acquired.

A number of factors can cause ligament sprains, including low-quality foot gear. Never race-walk or run in anything but high-grade shoes. Keep them in good condition and replace them as often as needed, usually every 750 miles or so of training. Hazards such as rocks and potholes in the terrain can cause you to twist your ankle or knee, leading to ligament sprains. Watch carefully for such hazards when you are running.

Also be aware of running routes that contain an angled surface, such as a beach or the side of a hill. If you run in one direction on these surfaces, you may develop functional short-leg syndrome, a common cause of leg and foot sprains. Run on level surfaces whenever possible. If you must run on uneven terrain, be sure to run in both directions to try to compensate for the slope. When running on school tracks, use the outside lanes. The inner lanes often contain uneven patches.

The ligament sprains most often linked to running are lateral sprains or ones on the outside of the ankle. Medial sprains, on the inside of the ankle, occur less frequently. The runner usually has to take a fall to injure the anterior and posterior cruciate ligaments on the inside of the knee. More common are sprains to the medial and lateral collateral ligaments, which are on both sides of the knee. We strongly recommend that you *avoid* the "hurdler's stretch," which can weaken the medial (inner) collateral ligaments of the knee. (The hurdler's stretch is a stretch where you sit on the ground with one leg straight in front of you and the other leg bent to the side and back behind you. You would then lean forward and touch your toes or your forehead to your kneecap.)

In some instances, the iliotibial band may be injured from running. This band, which attaches on the outside of the knee, stabilizes the knee immediately before and during the heel strike. As the iliotibial band moves from behind the thigh bone to the forward position, it may become inflamed. The irritated tissue then swells and becomes painful. In most cases, this condition will occur when you overstride, run downhill, or walk down stairs. A special stretching exercise described in Chapter 18 can be used along with RICE to treat this type of injury.

An ethyl chloride treatment can reduce the temperature and swelling of muscles, tendons, and ligaments, according to a series of experiments conducted by Hans Kraus, M.D., a sports medicine specialist. The ethyl chloride is sprayed on the injured area. The athlete then performs exercises that prevent the formation of adhesions and scar tissue. During the healing process, crutches are used to keep weight off the affected joints. According to Dr. Kraus, this method allows many injured people to resume their full athletic schedule within two weeks. Ethyl chloride spray must be obtained by prescription, however. If this is not feasible for you, the ice massage described previously may be used instead.

Chapter 8
▼

General Prevention and Treatment of Muscle, Tendon, and Ligament Injuries

Running itself rarely causes an injury. The problems usually stem from one of the many factors that contribute to your running approach, such as biomechanical problems with body structure, your running shoes, your warm-up and stretching routines, or the terrain on which you run. In short, most "running" problems are ones that you have allowed to develop. To prevent them, you must take better stock of yourself and your surroundings in relation to running.

Muscle injuries, for instance, commonly result from poor circulation and cold muscles, both of which can be avoided through a proper training program. The fatigue caused by daily activities and the local fatigue of specific muscle tissues also can lead to injuries. In addition, any anatomical problems with your body structure must be professionally evaluated and corrected.

The value of a warm-up prior to running and a cool-down afterward cannot be overstated. Of these two, however, the most important is post-exercise stretching. Your pre-running routine should be light, geared strictly at warming up the muscles and increasing their flexibility. Post-exercise stretching, on the other hand, must be comprehensive. Running tightens up the muscle fibers; therefore, they must be stretched back out to their full length when you have finished. Most people can get away with no pre-stretching at all, but everyone must take the time to stretch after a workout.

Be sure to include some range-of-motion exercises in your routine. A person's range will be limited if the muscles, joints, and tendons become inflexible or if scar tissue from an injury forms in the muscles and joints. A limited range of motion, in turn, puts you at a greater risk of injury. Your foot may strike the ground incorrectly, for example, if your shoulder muscle is tight and inflexible. Gentle, passive exercises, such as swimming, will help you maintain your full range of motion. Also the joint warm-up exercises and stretches discussed in Chapter 18 will give you a preventive effect.

Treatments in a flotation tank are one way to relax all the muscles. This procedure, which can both prevent and heal muscular injuries, can be done before or after exercising. If you do suffer a serious injury, allow the affected area adequate time to heal. The healing process will take roughly six weeks for the average person and somewhat longer, perhaps, for an older athlete. If you push too much when you first resume running, you could re-injure the area and create an even worse problem.

A well-designed program of "functional progressions" will provide you with a safe return to running following an injury. The progressions are a sequence of increasingly difficult workouts that gradually lead you back to your pre-injury running level. The program begins with exercises that strengthen and stretch tissues in the injured area. You then progress to a combination of walking and jogging. For several weeks, your training sessions should consist of the following sequence: Walk a specified distance, jog the distance, then walk it again. After that, step up the program to a jogging/running/jogging combination. Remember not to increase your speed, distance, or time by more than 10 percent every two weeks. In time, you will have returned to your normal schedule.

▼

Chapter 9

Bones and Skeletons

Anatomical bone structure plays a big role in running form and technique. The better that structure, the better the chances are that you will excel at running. Few of us are born with a perfect structure, however. Most people have genetic imperfections that must be accounted for in their running technique. Although these imperfections may keep you from becoming a first-class runner, they certainly will not prevent you from benefiting physically and spiritually from the experience of running.

To avoid running injuries, you must gain some understanding of the body parts most susceptible to injury. Improper bone structure or the malfunctioning of any body part can have a negative impact on your running form, particularly the way in which your heels strike the ground. As stated earlier, all the body parts are interdependent; the factors that affect one will also affect the others. What follows are the most common structural problems.

Metatarsus Adductus

The long bones on the top of the feet, called the metatarsals, stretch to each of the toes and account for nearly half of the bone structure in your feet. Many people are born with an abnormal positioning of these bones, called metatarsus adductus. The bones point inward, toward the center of the body, which improperly transmits the force of running and walking through your feet. Unfortunately, this disorder can only be corrected during a child's early formative years.

If you have this condition, you can minimize the effects by avoiding running shoes that are "C lasted," meaning the front portion of the shoes looks like the letter "C." (If you look at the

25

sole of your shoes, you will see that the portion that extends from the middle of your shoes to your toes is either straight, slightly curved in, or curved in greatly—in this case, C-lasted.) This type of shoe produces more discomfort in your feet and improperly transmits the shock of running through the feet and legs. It may lead to other problems if you try to shift the shock to other parts of the legs and body. The best protection is to wear straight-last shoes.

Excessive Pronation

This is another common congenital problem. The heel bones turn inward excessively, twisting the ankles inward and flattening the arch. You may have excessive pronation if your arches appear to be flat when you are standing or if your shoes collapse inward. If so, take the condition seriously. It can create problems all the way from your toes to your neck. Normal pronation increases three to four times during running; therefore, excessive pronation will do the same.

Orthotic devices can help position the feet so that they properly convey the force of running through the body. The devices also promote a proper range of motion, which helps to prevent injuries. The muscles and tendons of the feet and legs pull at the correct times and the correct angles. In some cases, prefabricated orthotics sold at athletic stores will serve the purpose. If the pronation is severe, however, a sports podiatrist can provide custom-made orthotics.

Short-Leg Syndrome

Nearly all cases of short-leg syndrome are functional in nature rather than congenital. A number of factors can create the functional imbalance, including a slanted running surface, unequally pronated feet, tight rear leg muscles, and/or an acquired pelvic imbalance. A small number of cases, roughly 5 to 10 percent, are structural problems in which a true congenital short leg or pelvic imbalance exists.

In either case, the short-leg syndrome can affect the foot, the back, or the neck, often on the side of the body opposite the shorter leg. The many injuries and problems that can result from the condition include ankle sprains, plantar fasciatis, heel spurs, knee and hip pain, stiff shoulders and neck, sciatica, lower back pain, and slipped discs.

In the few cases of congenital short-leg syndrome, a heel lift must be used at all times to create the proper balance. In all other cases, the source of the problem must be properly diagnosed to determine the correct treatment. As a preventative measure, try to run on level surfaces only. Or, at the very least, run in both directions on an angled surface to distribute the stress throughout the body. In addition, stretch lightly before running and heavily afterward to loosen and flex the rear leg muscles.

If you have a functional pelvic imbalance, a chiropractor, osteopath, or podiatrist can identify the problem. A kinesiologist, often a chiropractor, can teach you how to rebalance the pelvis through applied kinesiology, the science of muscular movements. These simple techniques can be used before or after running. However, they must be clinically taught and individualized for you. And finally, a podiatrist can make orthotics if they are needed.

Temporomandibular Joint Imbalance

A misalignment of this joint, located in the jaw, can produce a poor running form. It causes a strain on the neck muscles and vertebrae and strained breathing. By correcting the imbalance, running will put less stress on the body. This, in turn, will help to prevent injuries. One way to correct the problem is through a chiropractic adjustment of the temporomandibular joint (TMJ). If the adjustment holds for at least several months, then the method of treatment is adequate. If the joint continues to misalign, however, you may need to get a special TMJ device from a sports dentist trained in TMJ therapy.

A number of congenital deformities in the spine and legs can create problems for runners and decrease their efficiency. These structural abnormalities range from a curvature of the spine to being bow-legged or knock-kneed. Although none of these problems, even in severe cases, will prevent people from running, both their running technique and the intensity of their training must take the condition into consideration.

Your body posture, and thus your running ability, will be affected by a curvature of the spine. This condition, whether congenital or acquired, alters body movements and heel strike. To avoid injuries and enhance your ability to run long distances, try to adjust your posture and running form. Certain errors in your posture can be identified by having someone watch you or videotape you while you are running. In other cases, a chiropractor, osteopath, or orthopedic surgeon can identify and treat a spinal problem or injury. In some instances, the Alexander Technique may help to alleviate spinal problems. (The Alexander Technique involves retraining you in the way to sit, stand, and walk, as well as all body movement, which in turn helps you naturally elongate your spine and allows your vertebrae to fall into proper alignment.)

Most spinal injuries in runners occur in the middle (thoracic) lower spine regions (lumbar and sacral) according to Douglas Jackson, M.D., who has written a monograph on spine problems in *Prevention and Treatment of Running Injuries* by Robert D'Ambrosia, M.S., and David Dres, Jr., M.D. (Charles B. Slack, 1982). By contrast, cervical injuries rarely result from running. A number of steps can be taken to prevent and treat the more common types of spinal injuries. These include rest, lower-back stretches, and exercises to stretch the hamstrings and rear leg muscles, which will reduce the amount of stress on the lower back. In addition, bent-knee sit-ups will tighten the abdominal muscles and thereby support the lower back.

You can also reduce the stress on your lower back and assist in healing a spinal injury by swimming with a water skier's life belt around your waist. Or you can "run" in deep pool water while wearing a special vest. If you have a spinal abnormality, you may also need to wear certain orthotic devices and foot gear and get your pelvis rebalanced. With any lower-back problem, especially one that persists, be sure to get professional advice and an accurate diagnosis.

Bone and Stress Fractures

Running frequently causes stress fractures, whereas bone fractures due to an acute injury from running are much less common. The stress fractures take place most often in the metatarsals of the foot, the heel, the tibia, and the fibula; they occur less often in the femur and pelvis.

In *Prevention and Treatment of Running Injuries*, Dr. Angus McBride, Jr., defines stress fractures as a partial or complete fracture of the bone when it cannot withstand the nonviolent stress that is applied in a rhythmic, subthreshold manner. That means that the fracture can result from an overloading of the bone when you increase your running speed or distance too quickly.

Women suffer from stress fractures more often than men. This can be attributed both to hormonal imbalances and to women's greater tendency to develop osteoporosis. Women also tend to overtrain initially for sports and running, according to Mona Shangold, M.D., who has written a monograph on "Exercise in the Adult Female, Hormonal and Endocrine Effects," in *Exercise and Sports Science Review* (Volume 12, 1984).

Stress fractures account for 6 to 10 percent of all running injuries, according to "Injuries to Runners," an article by Dr. James Bates Ostering in the *American Journal of Sports Medicine* (1978). Nearly all of these fractures occur in the legs. This type of injury, in fact, is one of the few that will require you to stop running completely until the condition is healed. Although heat, rest, and massage can speed up the recovery rate, the bone will need about eight weeks to recover. Magnetic therapy has also been shown to greatly speed healing.

In most cases, a person can safely return to running by properly caring for the fracture and controlling any structural problems with orthotics and good foot gear. When you resume running, begin by cutting your pre-injury mileage in half. In the ensuing weeks, use functional progressions to return gradually to your usual running program. A safe way to recondition your bones and accustom them to the stress is to increase your running speed, duration, and intensity by 10 percent every two weeks.

Bursitis

When the tissue sacs in certain parts of the body become inflamed, they fill up with the lymph and synovial fluid created in the joints. Runners may get this condition, called bursitis, in the hips, knees, ankles, and the first and fifth metatarsals. An injury to a joint or to the tendons and ligaments surrounding a joint causes the bursitis. The body then tries to prevent motion by prompting the bursa to swell. The resulting muscle spasms will limit motion and create pain during movement.

In treating bursitis, you should immobilize the area to prevent any movement, the very goal that bursitis itself is intended to accomplish. With acute symptoms, the treatment should include RICE, passive range-of-motion exercises, and stretching exercises designed to stop the spasms. In cases where the swelling is severe, consult a doctor to determine if there has been a permanent thickening of the bursa tissues.

Physiotherapy can help you return to running safely. While many doctors use cortisone injections to reduce the swelling, this treatment can create other problems, such as weakened tissues and a greater chance of re-injury should the cortisone injections allow you to resume running too soon. In some cases of bursitis of the knee, the fluid may need to be professionally drained to reduce the inflammation and pain.

A related condition, called adventitious bursitis, occurs when the soft tissues around a bone become inflamed. In this case, there is no true bursa (tissue sac) present. Instead, as lymph fluid enters the affected area to soothe the joints, it is trapped by the soft tissue. The inflammation of the bone and its lining resembles a true bursitis, and the same treatment as for bursitis applies: Use RICE initially and protect the affected area. A combination of heat and massage can then be applied.

Bone bruises with bursitis typically occur in the metatarsals or the heel of the foot. When the bone is traumatized, such as when you trip on a pothole or a stone, the sudden impact adds to the trauma already created by running or walking. As a result, the lining of the bone becomes inflamed. This condition can take as long to heal as a complete fracture and create even more pain. Eight weeks is a typical recovery time. Again, the healing period should be followed by a gradual return to running.

Runner's Knee

This condition, chondromalacia patella, occurs when the articular surface of the kneecap is damaged. In some cases, the injury also affects the cartilage of the thigh bone. Potential causes include overstriding, a poor-grade running surface, and improper or poorly maintained running shoes. The symptoms include a clicking or noisy knee and extreme pain when running long distances, running on hills, and walking down stairs.

Another major cause of runner's knee is hypermobility (imbalance) of the foot. In this case, orthotic devices can prevent injuries and control the disorder. Avoid undergoing surgery to have the damaged cartilage "scraped." Instead, stick to conservative therapies and exercises geared at strengthening the anterior leg muscles and stretching the rear leg muscles.

Cartilage Damage

Most often, runners get cartilage damage in the knees, ankles, and metatarsals. The pain and swelling mimic the symptoms of bursitis. In most cases, people with cartilage damage can resume running in six to twelve weeks if they overcome the initial pain and resist a surgical treatment. To prevent this damage, wear shoes that fit properly, use orthotics when needed, and warm up the joint prior to running with gentle range-of-motion exercises.

In some cases, cartilage damage will be severe, especially in the knee. The cartilage tends to calcify and turn into bone. This, in turn, aggravates nearby joint tissues and cartilage, which may cause considerable discomfort when you run. Again, you should have such injuries diagnosed by a professional. But avoid a surgical solution if at all possible.

When the cartilage in a joint gradually wears away or becomes damaged, a related disorder called osteoarthritis may develop. Runners tend to get this condition faster than the general population because the activity stresses the cartilage. To prevent and minimize the damage, address any problems created by imperfect bone structure and excessive stress.

Chapter 10
▼

Skin

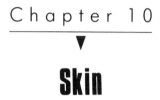

The various skin problems associated with running include blisters, sunburn, black toenails and fungus, and reactions to poisonous plants and insect bites. The appropriate treatments and preventative measures are as follows.

Blisters

Friction and pressure on the skin cause blisters, perhaps the most common of all running-related skin problems. The friction itself may be produced by ill-fitting socks and shoes and running surfaces that shift the foot from side to side, such as hills and running tracks. If you get blisters repeatedly, identify the causes and correct them.

Buy good running shoes that fit properly and break them in gradually. Make sure that your socks are not worn out, bunched up inside your shoes, or too tight. You may want to try socks made of materials that ease friction and help to prevent blisters. In addition, look for running surfaces that do not cause a tortional motion (twisting side to side) of the feet.

If you do get a blister, wash it off well with soap and water and then sterilize it with alcohol or an antiseptic. Sterilize a needle as well and puncture the side of the blister. If you just break the skin over the blister and allow the fluid to drain onto a sterile gauze pad, the procedure should not be painful. Do not remove the loose skin from the blister; it will act as a natural protective covering. At this point, cover the blister with a sterile dry gauze pad and some paper skin tape. Aloe vera and Vitamin E oil can add to faster healing.

In the course of a week, the skin over the blister will harden and peel. Protect the area until the skin is healed. When you run again, you may want to place moleskin over the blister. This inexpensive cotton padding, which adheres to the skin, will help to prevent a reblistering or irritation of the affected area. Always put a little cotton or gauze under the moleskin over the blister.

Sunburn

Runners often experience sunburn, particularly when the seasons change and they expose previously protected areas of the skin. As the sun becomes more intense, use a sunscreen with a protection rating of at least fifteen until your skin becomes accustomed to the exposure. You can then switch to a lower protection rating if desired, which allows more ultraviolet rays to reach the skin.

Fair-skinned people or those with a history of skin cancer, however, should use a sunblock with a rating of at least forty-five every time they are in the sun. Reapply as needed during long exposures. The risk of sunburn can also be reduced by taking Vitamin C and several hundred milligrams of PABA (paramenabenzoic acid) orally prior to any sun exposure.

Shoes that are too tight may cause the toenails to turn black suddenly. As stated earlier, your running shoes must include an extra inch of room at the front to allow the foot to move forward. If your shoes are too short, the toenail will hit the end repeatedly as you run. The trauma causes bleeding under the nails (the "blackness"), which can induce pain or become bacterially infected.

Fungus nails, by comparison, are characterized by an incremental thickening and darkening of your toenails. This condition may not cause any pain but will tend to be recurring because the fungus starts at the "root" of the nail. Contrary to popular belief, you don't contract fungi in the locker room. A fungus occurs naturally in different parts of the body, particularly in warm and moist areas. Thus, your feet are a prime candidate for this skin condition.

But even those external conditions are not enough to produce a fungus. If that were all it takes, everyone who worked out and sweated would develop fungus nails. The people who do develop fungi also have weak T cells, the portion of the immune system that fights all fungus invasions and many viral attacks. Such factors as stress and nutritional deficiencies can weaken T cells.

By keeping your feet as cool and dry as possible, you will eliminate the conditions that allow a fungus to grow. In the summer, wear socks made of cotton and polypropylene to keep perspiration away from the body. In the winter, switch to a wool/polypropylene combination. Another tactic is to alternate your running shoes each day to dry out the shoes and prolong their life. Foot powder can help keep your feet dry too.

Herbal salves and herbal solutions can be used to treat fungus infections on skin. (See Appendix A and B.) These natural methods can safely prevent an acute case of itching and blistering that may accompany the fungus. To apply the treatment, wrap your foot in sterile gauze bandage and saturate the gauze with the herbal solution. Let the gauze dry completely on the foot, which may take several hours. The drying process will draw out inflammation and dry up the blisters. Repeat this process daily before bedtime; complete the treatment by applying the herbal salve when you go to bed.

Remember that fungus infections also can develop in the groin area. In addition, running gear can irritate this skin and cause the same redness and itching as a fungus. If this occurs, replace the gear. If you develop a fungus, treat it promptly and then keep the area dry and cool to prevent another flare-up.

Poisonous Plants and Insect Bites

Steer clear of poisonous plants, such as poison ivy, when you run in the woods or a field. If you run in areas that may contain these plants, learn to recognize them and their seasonal changes. If you contact such plants with your pants, socks, and shoes, remember to remove them carefully to avoid getting the poisonous oils on your hands. Once it's on your hands, you could spread the contamination to other parts of your body. Remove your pants by holding the waist and turning them inside out as you peel them off. This will prevent any accidental contact with your legs.

If you get insect bites while running, use ice to control the itching and then apply Vitamin E oil and aloe vera to help heal the tissue. A stronger method, if needed, is to treat the area with an herbal tea solution. As with treating a fungus, wrap the affected area in sterile gauze and pour the tea onto the bandage. Allow it to dry naturally. As the tea evaporates, the inflammation and itching will subside. At bedtime, remove the bandage and apply an herbal salve. Use the salve two to four times a day until the skin has healed.

▼

Chapter 11

Genito-Urinary System

The genito-urinary system, which encompasses the genital and urinary organs, is susceptible to several conditions from running and exercise. Naturally, some of these conditions differ for men and women. Others, such as bladder disorders, can be experienced by either sex.

Bladder Conditions

Runners sometimes develop blood, myoglobin, or albumin in their urine. While the condition is often benign, it should be monitored by a doctor. Chronic symptoms could create more serious problems in the future. In many cases, unaccustomed strenuous exercise causes bladder problems. You may have blood in the urine when the body is dehydrated and the sides of the bladder rub against one another. This is yet another reason to drink plenty of water when you exercise.

Precautions for Women

Some women's bladders are positioned low in the body, which allows the organ to be jarred during running and puts them at risk for bladder disorders. To protect the organ as much as possible during a workout, be sure to empty your bladder before running. In addition, wear softer, shock-absorbent running shoes and train on a softer running surface. Another idea is to use replacement insoles that offer maximum shock absorbency.

Female runners also may develop menstrual irregularities, generally due to hormonal changes that take place during long-distance running. One study, however, showed that more than

90 percent of women who had regular menstrual functioning before running also were regular afterward. The ones who had menstruation problems after running had suffered from the same problems beforehand. Therefore, running alone was not to blame for oligmenorrhea or amenorrhea, in which menstruation decreases or stops. Studies have not yet determined, however, if such menstrual irregularities have permanent effects on the body.

Finally, women should wear a supportive, seamless bra made of natural fabrics when running. Although one study has shown that only one-fifth of women experience occasional breast pain while participating in sports, an inexpensive yet supportive bra can minimize jarring and help to prevent "drooping breasts," particularly in women with large breasts.

Precautions for Men

Male runners must wear either an athletic supporter or running shorts with a liner to support the genitalia. Avoid tight athletic supporters, which can cut off circulation and irritate the genitals. In addition, an insulated supporter or shorts may be needed to protect the testicles when running in cold weather.

The good news is that enlargement of the prostate, a common problem in aging men, occurs less often in runners than in the general population. However, conclusive research has not yet been conducted to show that the ability of long-distance running to improve the circulation helps deter such enlargement.

Chapter 12

▼

Respiratory System

Running earns the distinction of being an "aerobic" exercise because it promotes a series of events in the body that deliver large amounts of oxygen to the muscles. The process begins with the respiratory system, which delivers oxygen to the blood as you run. The blood then carries oxygen and fuel to millions of body cells. As the muscles burn this oxygen and release energy, they alternately tense and relax, a procedure that comprises the very substance of running and the definition of "aerobic" work.

For the muscles to receive this oxygen, the respiratory and circulatory systems must be able to deliver it to the blood. The process then works in reverse to eliminate such waste gases as carbon dioxide—the gases move from the muscles, to the blood, and then to the lungs, which release them from the body. Long-distance running makes this system of exchange more efficient, provided runners learn to breathe properly and to prevent damage from factors such as air pollution.

Proper Breathing

Few runners breathe well enough to make good use of their internal "exchange surface material," the 108-square-yard area in which gases pass back and forth between the blood and the lungs. For the most part, people breathe 23,000 times per day, or 16 times per minute. Via yoga breathing techniques, abdominal breathing techniques, and long-distance running, however, they could be exchanging more gases with each breath. As a result, they would require fewer breaths overall and reduce the stress on their respiratory system.

While most people breathe with their chest or thorax, the

abdomen produces the most efficient breathing. The stomach should expand slightly as you inhale and depress as you exhale, forcing air out. The rhythm should feel natural, not forced. Most good athletes use this technique because it exchanges gases more efficiently, produces more energy, and reduces fatigue.

Air Pollution

Undoubtedly, air pollution presents a serious problem for long-distance runners. In thirty minutes, a polluted urban environment can do the same damage as a half a pack of cigarettes in terms of putting carbon monoxide, carbon dioxide, and other toxins into the body. Whenever possible, run in parks during the daytime, when oxygen levels are high. Trees and grass provide the air with oxygen and remove waste products, thereby improving the relationship between good and bad gases. Conversely, avoid all polluted areas, particularly places that have a lot of automobile traffic.

Asthma and High-Altitude Pulmonary Edema

While asthma does not prevent its victims from running, neither does the condition improve due to a running program. Therefore, asthmatic people must be satisfied with the fact that they can perform as well as anyone else, using the proper medication when needed.

Exercise-induced asthma may have to be controlled by prescription medication to allow you to exercise. However, strengthening the immune system may stop this form of asthma completely.

High-altitude pulmonary edema often occurs when runners try to do "too much, too fast, too soon" at a high altitude. The initial symptoms include headaches, fatigue, nausea, and giddiness. A dry cough, difficult breathing, and chest pain may follow. This is a serious respiratory problem, and it should be avoided by letting your body become accustomed to a change in altitude slowly. Pay particular attention to this problem if you are vacationing in a high-altitude spot or returning to a high altitude following several weeks in a lower-altitude place.

Chapter 13
▼
Circulatory System

Good circulation is just as important to power walking and running as it is to your overall health. The circulatory system carries blood throughout the body, delivering the oxygen and nutrients needed to fuel body functioning. It also carries away waste products. When the circulatory system is in excellent condition, it allows the heart to operate more efficiently and, therefore, extends life.

Through proper training, runners can improve both circulation and heart functioning, which, in turn, makes it easier to run long distances. Running has a number of beneficial effects on the heart. It enhances the organ's strength, size, and efficiency. The carrying capacity of arteries and the number of arterioles (the smallest arteries) increases. Fatty deposits and hardening of the arteries also may be prevented, to some degree, by running.

A bigger and stronger heart lasts longer because it doesn't have to work as hard to get its job done. The well-conditioned heart pumps more blood with each beat; thus, it requires fewer beats to deliver blood to the body. Meanwhile, the carrying capacity of the entire circulatory system increases. A higher volume of blood flows through the body, increasing the count of red blood cells. This, in turn, improves the rate and volume of gas exchange in the body.

As the heart grows stronger from running, both the resting heart rate and the exercising rate will drop. A 60-second pulse count at the wrist or temple will measure the improvements in this area. Be sure to count for the full one minute. If you count for a few seconds and then multiply to reach 60 seconds, any beat you miss will be multiplied the same number of times. Hence, it could make a significant difference in the actual count.

The pulse count during exercise should stay within your "target range," the minimum and maximum heartbeat for an individual. The formula for determining a target range was discussed in Chapter 3, but it bears repeating here. You can only train properly by identifying your range and then staying within those parameters when you are exercising.

To determine the target range, begin by subtracting your age from the number 220. The result is a safe maximum for your heart; i.e., the heart should never exceed this number of beats per minute. According to many experts, a well-conditioned athlete can add 5 to 10 percent to this count because his or her heart works so efficiently. But for most people, even those in excellent shape, exceeding this maximum number could prove dangerous and increase the risk of a heart attack.

Therefore, the proper target range for an individual is 60 to 90 percent of the safe maximum number. To exercise safely and efficiently, you must stick to this range. If you exceed the 90 percent mark, the body cannot get oxygen to the muscles fast enough to meet the rigorous demands that you are placing on them. At this point, the exercise will cease to be aerobic.

Testing Heart Functioning

Before you begin a running program, see your doctor for a complete physical examination and an exercise stress test. If you have any hidden heart problems, they must be uncovered before you undertake any strenuous exercise. This step is particularly important for people with a history of heart trouble, those who have not exercised for a long time, and anyone over the age of thirty-five. On occasion, even comprehensive testing will not reveal a heart problem, and an athlete will die due to the condition. But in most cases, the detection of a heart disorder can save a person's life.

The cardiac physical should include the following elements:

1. A blood work-up. This will test liver and kidney functioning as well as levels of cholesterol, sugar, tryglycerides, and high-and low-density lipoproteins. Women also can be checked for anemia.

2. A resting electrocardiogram.

3. A cardiovascular stress test.

For people with special concerns about heart functioning, two other tests are available: A 24-hour halter monitor will gather and store information about your heart in a small computerized box worn at the waist. And an echocardiogram, which uses a safe ultrasound technology, can see inside your heart and identify any problems, such as damage to the valves.

For the most part, though, the cardiovascular stress test is used to identify any heart disorders that may harm an athlete. During this test, you will exercise on a treadmill or a stationary bike while your heart rate, heart functioning, and blood pressure are monitored. The test ends when you have reached your maximum level of safe exhaustion. Remember that you alone must decide when to stop, regardless of what anyone else in the room tells you.

In addition, a trained cardiologist should conduct the test and interpret the vital signs. In some cases, the test itself could prove too taxing or even, in rare instances, trigger a heart attack. A cardiologist can recognize and prevent such an occurrence. Most athletes should have a cardiovascular stress test every other year; people over the age of fifty and those with a history of heart trouble should be tested annually. In deciding where to have the test done, shop around for a mid-range price. Do not go for the highest or lowest fees.

In most cases, the test will give you a green light to begin a running program. Even so, you must monitor your heart rate daily to determine if strenuous exercise is advisable on any given day. The first step is to determine your normal resting pulse rate when you awaken in the morning. To do so, take your pulse before you get out of bed each day and keep a log of the results. On days when your resting rate is two to three beats above the norm, you should train less vigorously than usual. If it is five to six beats higher, you should probably avoid running that day. The extra beats indicate that your body is stressed. Running may only compound the problem.

On the days that you do run, be sure to increase the intensity of your workout slowly so that the heart rate can gradually climb to its peak. The progression from a resting rate to a maximum exercising rate should not be too sudden or dramatic. The process should be like adjusting a dimmer, not switching on a light. By turning up the heart rate slowly, you will not subject your body to excess stress. Pre-running exercises will get the heart beating easily and prepare it for a workout.

Pay attention to your heart when you are running. In time, you should know when you are too stressed by the way it feels. In these instances, take your pulse as you run. If the pulse has climbed higher than usual, ease up on your pace. When you are done running, remember to reduce your heart rate just as gradually as you increased it. With long-distance running, the cool-down period accounts for more heart attacks and problems than the actual run. You can't push the heart to its peak and then stop short. The process must be gradual.

Detraining and Overtraining

Be aware that a detraining effect takes place when you do not run for a week or more. In the first few days, cardiac output changes little. Only 1 to 2 percent of your conditioning is lost in the first week. In fact, a short layoff of a few days' duration can benefit the body by allowing it to rest, particularly if you have been injured. You may even run in better form when you resume training.

Within five to twelve days, however, cardiac output begins to decrease. If the layoff lasts for two or more weeks, it will take some time and effort to return to your peak level of conditioning. At the eight-week mark, you will have lost 80 to 100 percent of the effects of training.

Overtraining, at the other end of the spectrum, also should be avoided. This occurs when a runner reaches peak condition and then continues to train hard, eventually wearing away at the body. Possible signs of overtraining include constant soreness, a lethargic feeling, and a lack of motivation to exercise. In addition, rapid weight loss, loss of sleep, abnormal consumption of fluids, and irregular resting heart rate may indicate that you are overtraining. To spot these problems in the early stages, runners should monitor their post-running weight, hours of sleep, daily fluid intake, and morning heart rate.

Remember, too, that a brief rest from running can be beneficial. Training too little is always preferable to training too much. So if any of these early warning signs exist, slow down with your training and allow the body to recuperate. Nothing will come of an obsessive need to continue running despite a clear indication of overtraining.

Sports Anemia

Strenuous muscular exercise can cause a condition called sports anemia, which occurs frequently in long-distance runners, swimmers, and such athletes as boxers and football players who experience repeated trauma. The disorder is indicated by a hemoglobin count below 12 gm/dl in women and 14 gm/dl in men. In certain cases, such as when an athlete's performance is slipping, sports anemia may be found by your doctor with a simple blood test.

The following factors may cause or contribute to sports anemia: inadequate iron intake; a decrease in intestinal iron absorption; blood loss; increasing blood volume; intravascular hemolysis caused by heavy training (a breakdown of red blood cells in the arteries); trauma resulting in hemoglobinuria (blood in the urine); and inadequate dietary protein.

During the first two to three weeks of heavy training, in particular, a temporary anemia may occur. Oftentimes, sports anemia can be prevented by taking two grams of dietary protein for each kilogram of food you eat each day. The condition usually can be treated with iron supplements.

Chapter 14
▼
Gastrointestinal System

The role of proper nutrition in a running program will be discussed later in this book. It should be noted here, however, that what you eat and when you eat it in relation to your workout routine will determine whether you have gastrointestinal problems. You may get diarrhea, for example, if you eat foods that contain lactose or that are hard to digest before running.

Another running-related problem, intestinal cramps, occurs when you "swallow" air, which then passes from the stomach to the intestines and induces the cramps. Take charcoal capsules during the run to prevent or alleviate this problem. In other instances, runners may get cramps because the digestion of carbohydrates slows down during exercise, allowing fermentation to occur in the small intestines and release carbon dioxide gases. Again, use charcoal capsules if necessary. It's also a good idea to abstain from eating for five hours prior to performing aerobic exercises. If you run first thing in the morning, do not eat until after you finish your workout.

Chapter 15

▼

Endocrine System

The effects of diabetes, a disorder of the endocrine system, may be reduced through a running program. Many studies have found that diabetics require less insulin when they engage in long-distance running, for example. A diabetic must work with a doctor, of course, to monitor the disease throughout the exercise program. A sports medicine doctor can teach diabetics how to recognize the signs of an insulin reaction to running, what changes to look for in the blood sugar level, and what impact running will have on their insulin dosage. Diabetics should eat a small amount of carbohydrates two hours before they exercise.

Some men who train regularly may find an increase in sex drive due to hormonal changes. Unfortunately, overtraining may lead to a decreased sex drive. Balance is everything.

Women who overtrain may change their hormonal balances, leading to irregular menstruation, the absence of menstruation, difficulty in conceiving, and low birth weights.

Chapter 16

▼

Hyperthermia

Runners can suffer from five types of heat reaction, ranging from heat rash, the least severe, to heat stroke, a serious and often life-threatening condition. Therefore, you must become acutely aware of the factors that contribute to excessive sweating, dehydration, and the body's ability to regulate its own temperature and stay within a safe range. Indeed, healthy body temperature should never vary by more than one to two degrees Fahrenheit. Anything above or below this narrow range can lead to illness or death.

Over time, athletes can improve their thermoregulatory system, which monitors and controls internal body heat. A conditioned athlete begins to sweat rapidly when exercising, but the amount of perspiration is moderate throughout the workout period. A new athlete or one who's out of shape, on the other hand, does not sweat as quickly because the body takes longer to recognize the increasing heat and dispel it through perspiration. When this athlete finally breaks a sweat, he or she will perspire profusely.

For runners, oversweating is a danger sign. It can cause the body to lose too much water and become dehydrated. And the possible consequences of dehydration are severe: They range from weakness and hallucination to heat stroke, kidney damage, and even death. Hot and humid weather can cause even the fittest of athletes to become dehydrated. As a runner, you must be aware that the body fluids can run quite low if more water is lost than absorbed, even in cases where you are sweating only moderately. For this reason, you must hydrate yourself before, during, and after a workout, according to the method described later in this chapter.

The five types of heat reactions are discussed below. They are followed by a list of ways in which you can protect yourself from these conditions.

Heat Rash

This condition, often called "prickly heat," is the least severe of heat reactions. It can appear on any part of the body when the skin becomes irritated, dry, and inflamed. Preventive measures include using body cream and powder and wearing clothing made of cotton and other soft materials. In addition, be sure to build up your body's tolerance for heat gradually. .

Heat Cramps

This heat reaction results from profuse perspiring. The muscles cramp due to the loss of salts and potassium produced by the sweating. You can prevent this problem by eating a lot of fruits, vegetables, and other foods with high levels of natural salt and potassium. Do not use salt tablets, however. They are not nutritionally sound and may even be dangerous. Hydrate yourself by drinking plenty of water throughout your workout period.

Heat Fainting

This heat reaction occurs when dehydration reduces the blood volume. The blood becomes thicker, less mobile, and begins to "pool" in the legs and/or the skin. Due to the insufficient blood flow, the body heat does not dissipate and the brain does not receive enough blood; the blood pressure drops and you've fainted. To treat this condition, get the person to a cool place, get them to drink water, and elevate their feet and legs.

Heat Exhaustion

One step beyond fainting (which at least stops you from doing further damage) is heat exhaustion. With this life-threatening condition, the thermoregulatory and circulatory systems cannot meet the demands created by long-distance running. Body temperature shoots up to 101 to 104 degrees, sometimes higher. As a result, the heart rate increases and you will perspire less. Because this condition can lead to heat stroke, you should go to a hospital immediately for medical care.

Heat Stroke

This serious and life-threatening hyperthermic reaction evolves from an uncontrolled case of heat exhaustion. As the skin becomes hot and dry, the body temperature may soar to 108 degrees or higher. When this extreme temperature is reached, delirium, unconsciousness, a coma, brain damage, and even death can result. To control the acute reaction, the victim's body should be iced, immersed in cool water, exposed to air, and/or splashed with water and fanned. It also helps to get some water down the person's throat to rehydrate the body. Of course, the stroke victim must then be taken to the hospital.

Preventive Measures

Considering the potential severity of heat reactions and the amount of heat exposure incurred by runners, it pays to take the necessary precautions against these conditions. What follows are the many different ways in which you can protect yourself from hyperthermic reactions while running:

1. Drink small amounts of water throughout the day to hydrate yourself before, during, and after running. If you drink a few large doses instead, much of it will be eliminated because the cells cannot absorb it all at once. Begin hydrating in this manner a few days before a long run. Drink water every couple of hours, regardless of whether or not you are thirsty. This is especially important when you will run in hot and humid weather. Ordinarily, a marathon runner should consume at least 80 ounces of liquid per day. On hot days and for long runs, add one pint of water for every two miles to compensate for the fluids that will be lost through sweating.

2. Weigh yourself before and after exercising to gauge your water loss and determine how much fluid you need to drink. For every pound of body weight lost, drink two cups of water. It's important to monitor your weight when engaging in any strenuous exercise program. If you lose too much weight, the body is sending a danger signal. Heat exhaustion sets in at a 5 percent loss and hallucination at 7 percent. At a 10 percent loss, heat stroke is possible; at 20 percent, you are at great risk of dying.

3. Eat foods rich in natural salts to prevent the loss of soluble mineral salts, known as electrolytes, along with the body fluids. Symptoms similar to those of heat stroke may develop if you replace lost fluids without replacing these electrolytes, which include sodium, potassium, chlorine, magnesium, calcium, phosphorus, and sulfur.

4. Do not take salt tablets, which can cause water loss and lead to even more serious heart problems.

5. Allow your body to build up its tolerance by slowly increasing the amount of time you spend in the heat.

6. Avoid running at midday, when the sun and temperature are hottest. Run in the early morning or late afternoon instead.

7. Be sensible on especially hot days. Slow down and sweat less to prevent hyperthermic reactions. If you feel especially stressed and fatigued, stop running. The body may be telling you that it cannot properly regulate your internal temperature.

8. Learn to recognize your body's warning signs. If a heat reaction begins, you'll know to reduce your pace or stop running altogether.

9. Monitor your heart rate to keep it within your target range. If it exceeds the 90 percent maximum, you may already be suffering from a heat reaction or about to experience one.

10. In the summer, wear light-colored clothing, which absorbs less radiation from the sun.

11. Drink cold water to replace fluids most quickly in the body. Cold water takes only ten to twelve minutes to empty from the stomach into the intestine, where most water is absorbed. Warm water, by comparison, takes at least fifteen to twenty minutes to pass through the stomach. Avoid ice-cold water, however, which can shock the system.

12. Do not drink liquids with a high sugar content because they will delay the release of water from the stomach and

the absorption of water back into the body. The higher the sugar content, the more slowly a liquid will move through the system. Stick with a drink containing 2.5 percent or less sugar when the fluid is intended to hydrate the body and provide water.

13. Do not drink alcoholic or caffeinated beverages. They have a negative effect on the entire body and serve as a diuretic, prompting a rapid loss of water through urination.

14. As much as possible, run with a partner. If either of you suffers from a heat reaction, the other will be able to offer assistance. In some cases, your partner may recognize that something is wrong with you even before you know it yourself.

Although hyperthermic reactions occur most often in the summer, don't be fooled into complacency during the winter months. In an effort to keep warm, you may prompt oversweating and dehydration. Therefore, you must hydrate yourself and take other necessary precautions to protect yourself in the wintertime, too.

Chapter 17

▼

Hypothermia

A combination of cold air and exhaustion can cause the body to lose more heat than it generates. When this happens, the core temperature of the body drops and a condition called hypothermia results. Runners must be extremely sensitive to their environment to avoid this problem. You could suffer from hypothermia even when the air temperature exceeds freezing, for example, if the amount of wetness, windiness, and coldness create a dangerous mix.

Indeed, hypothermia can stem from any of four primary causes: cold, wetness, the windchill factor, and tiredness. The wetness may result from the body's inability to perspire properly or from the weather itself. The temperature, when extremely cold, can cause hypothermia on its own; in other cases, warmer temperatures can combine with the other factors to produce hypothermia. And finally, runners who are fatigued may fail to protect themselves from potential dangers.

A runner who suffers from hypothermia will experience increasingly dangerous stages of the condition as his or her core temperature begins to decline. A typical progression is as follows: The person shivers uncontrollably and sometimes violently. He has trouble using his hands and then loses muscular coordination. At this point, he may stumble, become sluggish in his thinking and speaking, and even get amnesia. If the body temperature drops further, the shivering subsides. The victim's muscles become rigid and cause erratic movements. He will speak incoherently and become irrational and confused. Finally, he will experience severe muscular rigidity and become semiconscious. When the body temperature falls below 80 degrees, the victim will be unconscious. Below 78 degrees, most victims die.

In addition to hypothermia, athletes who run in cold weather may experience chills, skin chapping, and frostbite. Take the necessary measures to prevent these conditions.

Frostbite

This hypothermic reaction takes place when a cold temperature prohibits circulation to the skin and body tissues, sometimes killing those tissues. In this way, frostbite can lead to the loss of an affected area. The hands and feet are especially susceptible to this condition.

You must immerse your entire body in warm (but not hot) water to treat frostbite. If possible, go home immediately or even to a doctor's office to make sure you can do so. If you stop off somewhere to treat the frostbite, the affected area will refreeze when you go back outside. The whole body immersion will provide the frozen part with much warmer blood. You can then seek medical care as soon as possible.

Chills and Chapping

Coldness and trapped perspiration together can create body chills, a relatively mild reaction. To prevent or alleviate the condition, open up some layers of your clothing when you begin to sweat. This will allow the perspiration and heat to evaporate. Do not run on windy days if you have just overcome this condition.

Chapping occurs when exposure to cold and wind causes the skin to flake and peel from the hands, face, and lips, all of which contain small amounts of moisture. Use moisturizers and sunscreens that contain no water to protect these parts of the body, and be sure to keep them dry before, during, and after running.

Preventive Measures

Of all the protective measures against hypothermia, the clothing that you wear while running will do the most to alleviate any danger. The best way to dress for cold-weather running is with many layers of light clothing, as opposed to a few heavy layers. Each successive layer will trap the air warmed by your body. In addition, you can release a buildup of heat and sweat by opening a few of the layers. This is crucial because the dryer you stay, the better. Sweat-drenched clothing can make you two hundred times colder than dry clothing.

A thermal cotton or Thermax garment should be worn closest to the skin. Follow this with a piece of clothing that you can open up if you become too warm. Finally, top off these layers with a woolen garment, which will allow perspiration to evaporate and keep external moisture out. Also remember that mittens will keep your hands warmer than gloves.

The length of time you're exposed to the cold will determine the degree of insulation needed for your hands and feet. Short exposures require that you heavily insulate these extremities.

Longer exposures, however, will require *less* insulation. In this case, you could decrease your core temperature and produce shivering with heavy layers of mittens and socks. When the hands and feet become a bit cold, the body will respond by generating and retaining some heat. Therefore, you should concentrate most of the insulation on your body for long-distance running.

In addition to dressing properly, you must stay dry when running in cold weather. Use rain gear when necessary and be aware of the direction of the wind. You should run into the wind at the start, even though it takes more effort. That way, the wind will be at your back on the return trip, when you are sweaty. Relative to you, the wind speed will be less and thus will create less of a chill. Finally, be sure to eat properly and drink a lot of water in small amounts to avoid dehydration. And, of course, stop running altogether if you become too cold.

Chapter 18
▼
The Holistic Workout

To perform well at any sport, you must focus not only on the actual event—such as a training run—but also on what you do before and after that event to enhance your exercise regimen. The actions that you take during these two stages will improve your athletic performance, reduce unnecessary stress and strain on the body, and go a long way toward preventing injuries.

The holistic workout presented here guides you through all three stages of an aerobic routine: the pre-run warm-up, the running itself, and the post-run stretching. Each stage includes exercises and techniques that serve a specific purpose, such as relaxing the body, warming up the muscles, and stretching them after running to prevent tightening. Together, the three stages provide you with a comprehensive approach to working out that will contribute to your total well-being.

The Pre-Run Routine

This stage consists of relaxing before you run and warming up the entire body to prepare for the impact of running. Over the years, studies have established a link between a proper warm-up routine and the reduction of injuries. The process of warming up saturates the muscles with blood and increases their elasticity. In this state, the muscles, tendons, and ligaments can withstand a greater amount of strain without becoming injured.

A number of changes take place in the body as you warm up the muscles and flex the joints. The strength and speed of muscle contractions improve, which allows them to perform their full range of motion. You also conserve energy—and therefore can exercise longer—because it takes less energy to produce the necessary movements. In addition, the blood becomes thinner and flows more easily. That means it can supply nutrients to the muscles more quickly and remove waste products such as lactic acid that may cause cramping.

In the end, these positive changes and many others can help to prevent a heart attack. According to several studies, as much as three-fourths of people who participated in strenuous exercise without warming up had abnormal cardiograph tracings. Hence, even healthy, conditioned people can put too much stress on the heart if they do not prepare adequately for a heavy workout.

To begin the pre-run routine, it's best to relax the mind and body by meditating or by practicing yoga breathing techniques. The following breathing exercise, for example, offers a simple and effective way to relax: Lie on your back or stand by a wall or a tree, with your hands resting on your lower abdomen. Close your eyes gently. Now, begin breathing in and out through your mouth. Take five to ten deep breaths, breathing slowly and in a relaxed manner without holding your breath or forcing the air out.

Once your body is relaxed, open your eyes extremely slowly, allowing up to two minutes to pass before they are completely open. This process will prevent light from hitting the retinas too suddenly, which, in turn, could cause all of the muscles and tendons to contract. Naturally, this type of contraction would ruin the effects of the breathing exercise. At this point, take your pulse count to get a pre-running, resting rate.

Next, warm up the major muscle groups by walking in place or by lying on your back and "bicycling" with your legs in the air for two to five minutes. In addition, people who have a problem-free heart can do sit-ups to warm up the muscles gently. Sit-ups maintain the core strength of the body and help to improve your posture and form while running. They also strengthen the abdominal muscles, which prevent the pelvis from tilting forward and incorrectly arching the lower back. They must be done correctly, however, or they could do more harm than good.

A conventional sit-up, for example, can lead to lower-back problems. This exercise emphasizes the hip flexor muscles, which allow the torso and legs to bend toward one another. When the psoas muscle (one of the hip flexor group) is strengthened, it becomes shorter. This, in turn, creates more curvature in the lower back. Unfortunately, bending your knees or having someone hold your feet in place while you do the sit-ups does not eliminate this problem.

A correct sit-up—often called a stomach crunch—focuses on the abdominal muscles instead. For people with weak stomach and leg muscles, it is performed as follows: Lie on your back with your knees bent and touching together and your feet flat on the floor. Rest your hands on your shoulders or fold your arms across your chest; do not put your hands behind your neck to pull yourself up. Now, lift your head and raise your shoulder blades *only a couple of inches* off the floor. Repeat this exercise as many times as you can. Eventually you will progress to the next level.

For people with reasonably strong stomach and leg muscles, exhale as you sit up a few inches. Be careful not to lift your shoulders more than 10 inches, however, or you will shift the focus to the hip flexor muscles, including the psoas muscle. Hold the position for 10 seconds and then slowly lower your shoulders back to the floor. Repeat the exercise 5 to 10 times. Once this has been accomplished, you should then be able to do normal bent-knee sit-ups.

Normal bent-knee sit-ups are done quickly. Always exhale going up and inhale coming down. Never let the back of your head touch the ground until you are finished. Remember, the purpose of these exercises is to warm up major muscle groups by using them in rhythmic movements. Although sit-ups look deceptively easy to perform, you should take it easy during the first week or so. Do anywhere from 10 to 20 repetitions until you feel discomfort from the strain. After the second week, you can gradually build up the number of repetitions.

The next phase of the pre-running routine is to loosen the joints from head to toe. This will activate the synovial fluids, which lubricate the joints and ligaments and help to protect them from being strained when you run. If you have arthritis or a joint injury, you may want to perform these exercises in a pool at first. The water's buoyancy will permit a greater range of pain-free motion.

What follows are exercises for each of the major joints. Again, they should be performed slowly and without force. Move the joints in a relaxed manner, using very little effort:

▶ Neck: Stand straight and let your head drop forward gently. Raise it straight up again and then let it fall backward. Repeat the movement 10 times in each direction. Next, look to the left, then straight ahead, and then to the right. Repeat 10 times each.

▶ Shoulders: Hold one hand straight out in front of you. Move the arm around in a complete circle, 10 times forward and 10 times backward. Do not hold your arm too rigidly; focus on achieving a full range of motion. Repeat the exercise for the other arm.

▶ Elbows: Hold your hands in front of you, palms facing up, as if you were lifting a pair of dumbbells. Moving both elbows at once, curl your arms toward your body, and then lower them in a relaxed manner. Repeat 10 times. Do the exercise another 10 times with your palms facing downward.

► Wrists: Clasp the hands in a praying position and then gently move them from left to right, bending the wrists back and forth. The wrists should bend back on themselves softly. Repeat 10 times in each direction. Next, grasp your left wrist with your right hand and rotate the left hand in a circle. Keep the wrist relaxed and pretend to draw a circle with your index finger. Complete the circle 10 times clockwise and 10 times counterclockwise. Repeat the exercise with the other wrist.

► Fingers: Make a soft, relaxed fist with each hand, simply allowing the fingers to fold into your palms. Open and close both hands in a gentle fist 10 times. Next, spread your fingers wide apart on each hand and then close them slowly. Repeat 10 times.

► Hips: Stand with your feet shoulder-width apart. Rotate your hips in a slow and gentle circle, as if you are using a hula hoop. Repeat 10 times in one direction and 10 in the other.

► Knees: Stand with your ankles, feet and knees touching. Bend slightly forward at the knees, but not very deeply. Place your hands on top of your kneecaps and rotate them in a slow circle. Move your buttocks and knees together, 10 times clockwise and 10 times counterclockwise. Pretend that a pen extends straight out from your kneecaps and that you are trying to draw a circle with it.

► Ankles: Sit on a chair or on the floor and place your left ankle on top of your right knee. Hold your left leg just above the ankle with your left hand. Then use your right hand to grasp your left foot by the toes and rotate the foot. Keep the ankle loose and let your hand do the work. Never rotate the ankle by using your leg muscles. Rotate 10 times in each direction. Repeat with the other ankle.

► Metatarsals: Use your right hand to grasp the ball of your left foot. Flex the metatarsal joints (which stretch from the toes to the top of the foot) straight up and down 10 times, mimicking the motion of walking. Then do the same for each toe individually. Switch and repeat with the right foot and toes. In addition, spend a few minutes massaging the top and bottom of each foot. The massage will stimulate the circulation to your feet, which absorb the greatest amount of shock from running. Using your fingers and palms, knead your feet in a circular motion, applying gentle pressure.

Once the joints have been loosened, you're ready to do some pre-run stretching. Remember that these exercises must follow the warm-up routine because stretching cold muscles can promote injury. The focus before running is on passive stretching— a relaxed and gentle extension of the muscles to enhance flexibility. "Ballistic" stretching, on the other hand, should be avoided. It includes a bouncing motion as you enter the extension. These exercises tighten, rather than loosen, muscles and tendons. They also may tear tight muscles.

With the passive stretches described here, you perform a continuous stretching motion and then hold the end position for anywhere from 10 to 30 seconds. Try to control the extension with your hands and arms rather than with your body weight. This will make you more aware of the length of the stretch. Finally, remember that more stretching is not necessarily better. You should be as relaxed as possible when performing these exercises:

► Quadriceps: Perform this exercise with each leg to stretch the quadricep muscles in the front of the thighs. Place your right hand against a wall to brace yourself. Grasp the top of your left foot with your left hand. Then pull your foot up behind you until it touches your buttock. Make sure the foot is aligned straight behind you, not twisted to the side. And be sure to keep the left thigh in front of the right thigh, never even with it. Hold the position for 20 seconds, pulling gently. Return the foot to the floor. Repeat 5 times for each leg if you ski or ride a bike; 2 to 3 times if you participate in any other sport. This exercise also can be performed while lying on your side.

▶ Buttocks and Hamstrings: The "kiss the knee" stretch will alleviate stress on the lower back and help to stretch the upper rear leg muscles. Again, it should not cause pain. Slow down if you feel any strain on your legs or back. Lie on the floor and bend your right knee. Place both hands behind the knee. (Never put our hands on top of your knee; they may slip and cause the kneecap to jam into the thigh bone.) Pull your knee toward your chest and lift your head slightly, as if you were going to kiss your knee. Hold the position for 20 seconds. Lower your foot and leg completely to the floor and then repeat the stretch 5 times for each leg.

▶ Lower Legs and Feet: This exercise, called the "towel stretch," will stretch the lower rear leg muscles, the Achilles tendon, and the gastrochemius and soleus muscles. The exercise should not be painful; if it does cause discomfort, be even more gentle with your execution. To begin, get a towel or belt. Sit on the floor with your legs extended straight out in front of you and your feet pointing up. Sling the towel around the bottom of your right foot, holding the ends of the towel in each hand. Lean back slowly toward the floor, keeping your legs relaxed, your heels on the floor, and your back straight.

This motion will automatically pull your foot toward your face. Let your upper-body weight do the work, not any additional muscle power. Hold the position for 20 seconds, keeping your foot as loose as possible. You can test how relaxed you are by letting go of the towel with your right hand. Your right foot should spring forward to the same position as your left foot if the leg is really relaxed. Repeat the stretch 3 to 5 times for each leg.

The Run

This stage of your workout consists of two distinct phases. The first requires you to visualize yourself as you will look when you run and practice the essential motions. The second brings you to the aerobic workout itself.

During the visualization phase, spend a few minutes drawing a mental picture of yourself as a long-distance runner. Now is not the time to be modest. In this picture, which you alone control, you have excellent form and technique, and you are performing the run perfectly. This type of imaging and psychological rehearsal can do a great deal to enhance your performance in any sport, whether it be running, skiing, or swimming. In essence, you must recognize the link between the mental and physical worlds: Images of a well-executed run can influence your actual performance, just as the thoughts of eating something sour can make you salivate.

Next, you are ready to act out the exact motions that you will use to perform the run. This routine will warm up the specific muscles to be used and prepare them for the stress that they are about to endure in performing those very movements. The technique is akin to shadowboxing. You simply go through all of the motions without actually running. (For other sports, you pretend to swing a racket, bicycle with your legs, etc.)

At this point, just before the run, take time to practice an alternative breathing technique: Breathe deeply through your mouth and exhale slowly through your mouth. (You can get an even deeper breath by raising your arms to shoulder height while inhaling. Return them to your sides while exhaling.) Next, take a shallow breath in and out through your mouth. Repeat the two steps three times.

Keep in mind that your body will require plenty of oxygen during any extended period of aerobic exercise. You also need to release carbon dioxide by exhaling. Therefore, never hold your breath while exercising. This will only put pressure on your heart and reduce the amount of oxygen supplied to the muscles. Abdominal breathing—in and out through the mouth—is the best technique for aerobic workouts. If you breathe through the nose instead, you take in less air.

Now you're ready for the second phase—the actual running itself. You may be eager to move out fast, but that technique will only shock the system and place undue stress on the heart. Instead, begin the run by building up your speed slowly. The body takes eight to ten minutes to progress from an anaerobic to an aerobic state, so be especially careful during the first ten minutes of your run. It's simply a bad idea to go too fast during this initial period.

Next, do a mental check of your running form. Your back should be straight, with your body bent forward just slightly. Your head should be level, not looking down at your feet. And your arms should be bent, swinging gently forward and backward just at your waistline. Keep your hands relaxed with your fingers gently closed. To cushion the impact of running on your body, make sure that you hit the ground toward the back of your foot; then roll the foot from heel to toe.

As this point, another visualization technique can reduce the amount of stress on your system. Imagine that you are floating and barely touching the ground. This mental image will help you to keep a light touch and avoid a bouncing or jarring rhythm. Your head should move up and down only slightly. Your landing should be a soft and gentle roll that promotes an even gait.

You can also prevent jarring effects on the body by running on grass and earth, such as on a golf course or along a wooded trail. Since this is not always possible, try to run on asphalt as opposed to concrete roads. Take the condition of the road into consideration, too. In many cases, the shoulders of a road are lower than the center and slightly angled. Since in order to be safe you must run facing traffic, your left leg will land on a lower surface. This could cause various imbalances in your torso and legs. To prevent these imbalances, run on a flatter road or a less traveled one where you can switch to the right side as well, somewhat evening out the effects of the angled running surface.

Running tracks have their good and bad points. Although an indoor track offers a cushioned surface and a consistent climate, it can become monotonous if the track is small. In some cases, a short circumference could even create problems with lateral torque. Likewise, outdoor tracks can be boring for the runner and create certain structural imbalances. Be sure to run in both directions on such tracks to distribute the effects of a sloped or uneven surface equally throughout the body.

The Post-Run Routine

This stage of the aerobic workout consists of a comprehensive stretching routine to alleviate tightening of the muscles and a cool-down period in which your heart returns to its resting rate.

Post-run stretching is a critical element in a running program. The loose and limber feeling we have right after exercising is deceptive. Any strenuous use of the muscles, tendons, and ligaments makes them tighten up; hence, they must be stretched out to their pre-running length to prevent injuries. The proper amount of stretching will depend on your individual needs. It could take anywhere from 10 to 30 minutes to complete the routine. If you're not stretching sufficiently, you'll know it the next day because the muscles will feel tight.

Each of the stretches presented here should be repeated 3 to 5 times, holding the extension for 20 to 30 seconds. As with the pre-run routine, these exercises must be done gently. Move smoothly into the extension and reach for your limit. Don't ignore any signs of strain from your body. And don't hold your breath as you stretch. Keep breathing regularly as you perform the exercises.

Following are five basic stretches for the rear leg muscles, mid-calf muscles, hamstrings and buttocks, quadriceps and inner thighs, and groin:

▶ Rear Leg Muscles: Stand facing a wall as closely as possible, with your feet and body almost touching it. Position your feet about shoulder-width apart. Place the palms of your hands flat against the wall, at about face level or higher. Take a step back with the leg to be stretched. Keep the leg in a straight line with the rest of the body and still shoulder-width apart. The front knee will be bent at about a 90-degree angle. Lean forward to stretch the back leg, supporting yourself with your hands and forearms. Keep your back knee straight, your front knee bent.

At this point, your elbows should be against the wall, with your face looking between them. You should feel the stretch in your lower rear leg, up to the point just above the knee. Be careful not to hyperextend the knee by throwing your hips too far forward. In the beginning, you may want to check the positioning of your back leg. For the best stretch, your foot should be positioned at the point where your heel will just stay on the ground when you lean forward.

Finish the stretch by pushing out with your hands and moving your foot back slightly to the next farthest point that it will stay on the ground. This stretches the muscles a bit more, allowing you to repeat the exercise with your leg positioned farther back. If your heel rises up when you lean forward, move your foot slightly closer to the wall. Repeat the stretch 5 times on the first leg and then switch to the other leg.

▶ Mid-Calf: Repeat the first exercise with one basic variation: When you position the back leg, bend it slightly forward at the knee to stretch the soleus muscle in the mid-calf. Hold the extension for 20 seconds. Repeat the stretch 5 times in a row for each leg. Keep in mind that the angle of the stretch will be greater if you are wearing running shoes, which give you a mechanical advantage. Don't be confused if when you stretch at home barefooted, you cannot take as big a step backward.

▶ Hamstrings and buttocks: When the large muscles in the back of your upper legs get tight, they can exert pressure on your back and lead to injury. Tight hamstrings can also shorten your stride considerably, creating knee pain and other problems. Therefore, it's especially important to stretch the hamstrings after running.

To perform a safe hamstring stretch, begin by lying on your back. Raise one leg in the air and put your hands around the calf muscles. Pull your knee toward your forehead, but do not lift your head off the ground. You must keep your leg straight. Depending on the angle, the stretch will affect different parts of the hamstring muscle. Hold the extension for 20 seconds and then slowly lower your leg. Repeat the stretch 3 to 5 times for each leg.

▶ Quadriceps: To stretch the quadricep muscles in the front of the thighs, lie on the ground on your stomach. Bend one knee toward your buttock, then reach behind you with both hands to grasp the ankle. Press your heel down toward your buttock, holding the extension for 20 seconds. Switch to the opposite leg and repeat the exercise. If you are pressed for time after you finish your run, the standing-quadricep stretch described in the Pre-Run Section can be used instead. This time, keep both thighs even.

▶ Groin: The following exercise will stretch the inner thighs and groin area. Sit on the floor, bend both knees outward, and put the soles of your feet together. Position both hands on your ankles and use your elbows to apply a continuous pressure on the knees. Do not bounce your legs; simply try to get the outside of your knees to touch the ground. Hold the extension for 20 seconds and then bring your knees together. Repeat the exercise 5 times.

▶ Iliotibial Band: This stretch is used when the ligament that stabilizes the knee, the iliotibial band, becomes inflamed. Runners who have no symptoms of iliotibial band syndrome can skip this exercise. To begin, stand with one shoulder against a wall, then step away from the wall with both feet. Now cross your feet and let your hips curve gently toward the wall so that your body looks like the letter "C" in reverse. Switch shoulders and repeat the stretch for the other knee. Do the exercise 3 to 5 times per leg, depending on the amount of stiffness.

Once these post-running stretches have been performed, it's time to conclude the aerobic routine by cooling down the body and the heart rate. Most important, the blood that has flowed to your extremities while you were exercising must now be returned to the heart. That means you must keep moving until your heart rate is within twenty beats or so of its normal resting rate. In this way, the muscles will do the work of getting blood

65

back to the heart. The veins that deliver blood from the muscles to the heart cannot perform this function independently because they do not have their own pumping mechanism.

Once your heart rate has slowed down sufficiently, you can begin to relax, meditate, and stretch. The cool-down period should also be used to begin rehydrating yourself by drinking liquids. Do not, however, take a hot shower, sauna, or whirlpool right after a strenuous workout. The heat will cause the heart to work harder as blood is carried away from vital organs such as the heart and brain to the skin.

Finally, take time to fill out the log sheet presented in Appendix C. This fourteen-day log, which you can reproduce and keep in a notebook, allows you to record the various factors that influence your exercise each day. Don't limit yourself to comments about your physical condition; include any comments you may have on mental, spiritual, emotional, social, and economical factors as well. When exercising and training become a part of your daily routine, you will see that the log begins to serve as an ongoing commentary on many aspects of your life, not exercising alone.

Chapter 19
▼
A 28-Day Plan for Runners

At this point, you may be coming up with all manner of excuses for excluding an exercise program from your daily routine, but now is the time to make a commitment to improving your health. Once you recognize the importance of exercise to your well-being, you can structure a program that allows you to execute the workout safely and efficiently. This program will become an integral part of your life that contributes to your health each and every day.

Here we present a basic program called the "28-Day Plan for

Runners," which everyone can incorporate into a busy schedule. It includes the three stages of an aerobic workout discussed in the previous chapter: the pre-run routine, the running itself, and the post-run routine. During the plan's four seven-day cycles, you will run (or choose an alternative aerobic exercise) on Days 1, 3, and 5. Any day of the week may be designated as Day 1 of the plan; the sequence is the key.

For the first four weeks, you perform the aerobic part of the plan for twenty minutes each on Days 1, 3, and 5. Every two weeks after that, you increase the duration of the aerobic exercise by 10 percent, provided that you have no heart problems and are under thirty-five years of age. If you are over thirty-five or have a history of heart trouble, step up the length of the aerobic routine by 10 percent every four weeks instead.

Remember that the exercise plan is meant to serve as a guideline, not a rigid set of rules to be followed without variation. In choosing an aerobic exercise for Days 1, 3, and 5, consider your exercise goals, your strengths and weaknesses, and your lifestyle. Then choose an exercise that both interests you and meets the requirements of an aerobic workout (twenty to sixty minutes of exercise at your target heart rate).

One approach would be to rotate two complementary types of aerobic exercise, such as running and biking. Both will strengthen leg muscles while improving your aerobic conditioning. Depending on the weather and other factors, you simply choose one or the other on your "aerobic days." You could run outdoors, for example, and ride a stationary bike indoors, thereby accounting for all seasons. Swimming, which can be conducted indoors or out, would be another complementary exercise.

Your best time for exercising may be in the morning, at noon, or at night. To determine when an exercise regimen feels best, you must be in tune with your body. Learn to recognize the monthly cycles that influence your physical energy, your moods, and your intellect. Then build a routine into your schedule that accommodates those cycles and stick with it in your execution. Many people, for example, are most flexible at the end of the workday. For them, late-afternoon exercising would put that flexibility to use, reduce the tensions of the day, and help overcome the general fatigue caused by working.

Before you begin the program, make sure that you have properly prepared for the onset of strenuous exercise. All new runners should get a physical examination. Those who are over thirty-five or have a history of heart disorders also must take a cardiovascular stress test to identify any undetected heart problems. It's smart to obtain medical clearance. In addition, make sure that you have good running shoes that fit correctly.

The necessity of starting out slowly bears repeating here. Don't overdo it in the beginning, no matter how eager you are to get in shape. Take it slow until your body adapts. Remember that "too much, too fast, too soon" will likely lead to injury and set you back in your program. Many people, in fact, have a hard time returning to running once they are injured. Be sensitive to the small clues and messages your body sends you. If you feel especially tired on one of your aerobic days, cut the intensity and duration of your workout by half.

Now you are ready to put the 28-Day Plan into motion. Two variations of the basic plan are offered for people who want to include anaerobic exercises (i.e., sprinting for one to two minutes) in their workout routine and those who want to achieve above-average endurance and speed. Option A allows for the inclusion of anaerobic exercise or sports; Option B adds "interval training" to the basic aerobic plan.

The three stages of this exercise plan are discussed in detail in Chapter 18. To summarize, the "pre-run routine" includes relaxation, warm-ups for the entire body, joint flexing, and pre-exercise stretching. Next comes the "running," which is preceded by visualization techniques. And finally, the "post-run routine" includes stretching exercises and a cool-down period.

All seven days of the workout cycle include the pre-and post-run routines. Never skip these exercises unless you are ill. They are the foundation that will keep you healthy, flexible, and functioning properly. The only variable is the running stage (or other form of aerobic exercise), which takes place on three of the seven days and may change depending on your needs and interests.

Perform the following seven-day routine four times to complete the 28-day cycle. The aerobic exercise lasts for 20 minutes during the first cycle. On Day 1 of the fifth week, add 10 percent to the time spent exercising aerobically; i.e., the exercise lasts for 22 minutes.

DAY	STAGES	TIME
1	The complete aerobic routine: pre-run; running (or other aerobic exercise); post-run	20 min.
2	Pre-run and post-run routines	
3	The complete aerobic routine	20 min.
4	Pre-run and post-run routines	
5	The complete aerobic routine	20 min.
6	Pre-run and post-run routines	
7	Pre-run and post-run routines	

Every two weeks, add 10 percent to the aerobic exercising time period until you have reached the following time limits for each type of exercise:

EXERCISE	TIME LIMIT
Running	30 minutes (for non-competing athletes)
Walking	1 ½ hours
Swimming	45 minutes to 1 hour
Bicycling	30 minutes (for non-competing athletes)
Jumping (with or without a jump rope)	30 minutes (do not exceed this limit with jumping due to its intensity)

Take your pulse rate throughout the aerobic period to ensure that it is within your target range (60 to 90 percent of your maximum safe rate). As your physical conditioning improves, it will take more effort to reach and maintain your target rate. Keep working harder until you have reached the time limits defined above for each type of exercising. If you wish to go beyond those limits, increase them according to the amount of time that it takes to reach and sustain your target heart rate.

Remember that the Basic 28-Day Plan can be used all of your life. On your birthday each year, you simply recalculate your target heart rate by subtracting your age from the number 220 and then setting the range at 60 to 90 percent of that maximum number. To make the plan more demanding, you can perform the aerobic exercise on four days instead of three. Day 6 or 7 would be a good day on which to add more aerobics to the basic plan. When training for a marathon, you may want to alter the schedule as follows: Train three days, rest one, train three days, etc.

Option A

This variation of the basic plan accommodates those who want to alternate an anaerobic exercise with the aerobic workout. While you can achieve and maintain good conditioning with the basic plan, Option A allows you to do even more. The anaerobic exercises could include such sports as tennis and golfing or weight training and calisthenics.

Option A includes the anaerobic exercise or sport on Days 2 and 5. You must allow forty-eight hours between periods of anaerobic exercise because the intensity of the workout breaks down tissues. Therefore, it takes forty-eight hours for the body to rebound and repair any damage. Those who choose to do calisthenics (such as push-ups, sit-ups, and jumping jacks) must be careful to perform the exercises correctly. Sloppiness will only tire you out. And when you're tired, you're more likely to quit or get injured.

With Option A, you follow the Basic 28-Day Plan for the first four weeks. The chart below begins on Day 1 of Week 5. On Days

1 and 3, you perform the aerobic exercise for 22 minutes. On Days 2 and 5, you perform the anaerobic exercise instead.

DAY	STAGES	TIME
1	The complete aerobic routine: pre-run; running (or other aerobic exercise); post-run	22 min.
2	The complete *anaerobic* routine	
3	The complete aerobic routine	22 min.
4	Pre-run and post-run routines	
5	The complete *anaerobic* routine	
6	Pre-run and post-run routines	
7	Pre-run and post-run routines	

Repeat this exact schedule during Week 6. For Weeks 7 and 8, increase the aerobic time period on Days 1 and 3 by 10 percent to a total of 24 minutes. Continue to alternate the aerobic and anaerobic exercises as shown in the schedule above. At the beginning of Week 9, increase the aerobic exercise period by another 10 percent to a total of 26 minutes. (If you are over age thirty-five or have a history of heart trouble, stay at 24 minutes during Weeks 9 and 10.)

For a particularly strenuous workout, you can perform both anaerobic and aerobic exercises on the same day. But they must be done in the proper order. Anaerobic exercises should never follow aerobic work because they limit the body's ability to recover from the stress and strain. Do it the other way around, with aerobic work following the anaerobic exercise. It's okay to go swimming, for example, after you play a game of golf or lift weights.

Option B

With this variation, you add a fourth day of running and one or two days of "interval training" to your aerobic workout. Again, this will take you a step beyond the good level of fitness provided by the Basic 28-Day Plan. Your stamina, endurance, and cardiovascular conditioning all will improve as you strive for excellence.

Interval training is an anaerobic exercise, so all of the precautions for Option A apply to this routine. It can be done with any type of aerobic work. When running, for example, the interval training takes place as follows: Run at your target heart rate for 10 minutes. Next, run to get your pulse count as close as possible to your maximum heart rate for 30 seconds; i.e., 90 percent of the maximum number. Then "rest" by running at your target rate for another 30 seconds. Repeat the sequence—a 30-second sprint, followed by a 30-second "rest"—four consecutive times during one aerobic exercise period. Add one repetition every month until you have reached a maximum of 10 repetitions.

We recommend that you perform interval training only one day a week. People with heart disease or another serious problem should only do this training with a doctor's supervision. It is intense work that can lead to injuries. It also requires a 48-hour recovery period, just as anaerobic exercise does. For most people, four 60-second sets of sprinting and resting (30 seconds each) will tire the body.

If you have set high conditioning goals, you may want to perform fitness training twice a week. In the schedule that follows, we allow for the training on Days 3 and 6 to illustrate the best spacing should you choose to do two days of interval training. This schedule begins on Day 1 of Week 5, when the aerobic exercise period has reached 22 minutes. Repeat the schedule for Week 6; then add 10 minutes every two weeks to the aerobic exercise period until you have reached 30 minutes of running (or the other time limits for aerobic exercises defined earlier in this chapter).

DAY	STAGES	TIME
1	The complete aerobic routine: pre-run; running (or other aerobic exercise); post-run	22 min.
2	Pre-run and post-run routines	
3	The complete aerobic routine, with *interval training*	22 min.
4	Pre-run and post-run routines	
5	The complete aerobic routine	22 min.
6	The complete aerobic routine, with *interval training*	22 min.
7	Pre-run and post-run routine	

A final word of caution: Do not add both Option A and Option B to the Basic 28-Day Plan. The body would not have sufficient time to recover from the stress of anaerobic work on one day and interval training on the next. To add that much strenuous work to the schedule, you would need professional guidance.

Chapter 20

▼

Healers and Therapies

It's not a foregone conclusion, by any means, that a runner will continuously suffer from injuries. As discussed in previous chapters, there are many ways in which you can reduce your chances of getting hurt. As a highly active person, however, there may be times when you experience some type of injury or pain. On those occasions, the most important course of action is to get an accurate diagnosis of the injury and good advice on the therapies that can be used to treat it. Here, we guide you to the types of healers who can provide that diagnosis and to the wide range of therapies available.

A professional diagnosis is critical to the healing process. Indeed, you should never try to diagnose an injury yourself. To begin to heal properly, you must know exactly what parts of the body are affected and the injury's level of seriousness. To locate someone to diagnose the problem, ask a trusted doctor and your relatives and friends for their recommendations. If necessary, travel a bit to reach a skilled doctor. It's usually worth the time and effort because a misdiagnosis can end up costing you in many ways.

Once the diagnosis has been made, you can work with the doctor to determine how best to treat the problem. You may follow the diagnoser's suggestion on what type of therapy to use, find alternative therapies, or use some combination of the two approaches. Traditional medical doctors, for example, may be great for diagnosing an injury but not necessarily for treatment because they tend to focus on the use of medications, injections, and surgery. In that case, you may want to explore some alternative therapies instead.

A number of factors will affect your decision about which healer and what type of therapy to use. These include the therapy's availability and cost, whether your insurance covers the therapy, the total number of treatments needed, and the amount of time each treatment takes. The healing method's possible risks and side effects must be considered as well. In many cases, you may want to combine two or more types of therapies to speed your recovery.

Remember that the easiest route may not necessarily lead to the best results. When choosing a healing professional, try to determine whether the person is truly caring, highly knowledgeable about the methodology, and willing to explain the procedures to you. In addition, he or she should be willing to work with other therapists as part of a "healing team" to help you recover.

While many healers do their jobs quite well, those with the characteristics described above will help you to heal faster. It's been said that a person to truly love is hard to find, but a fine healer is even harder! Don't worry, however. There are many shining stars in the world of therapy, so there is no reason to settle for second-rate care. It's *your* body that's being treated, and you have a right to expect the best.

Diagnosers

The following professionals can diagnose an injury and offer various forms of treatment:

Chiropractors: These healers "manipulate" the spine and pelvis to realign your bones and joints and return them to a normal position. They may use a variety of techniques, both gentle and forceful, to achieve the realignment. When the upper body is put into proper alignment and kept that way with various exercises, musculoskeletal injuries can heal. Chiropractors may aid the healing process with massage, heat treatments, and various physiotherapy devices.

Orthopedic Surgeons: These doctors specialize in treating diseases and injuries of the bones, muscles, tendons, and ligaments with medical and surgical approaches. They excel at diagnosing injuries. In most cases, however, they will recommend injections or surgery as the solution to your problem. You could find a surgeon, of course, who also has an interest in rehabilitation techniques and recommends that you try therapy first. But if the doctor is less committed to rehabilitation than to surgery, the therapy may be more likely to fail. This could lead right back to the surgical solution; i.e., "I'm sorry rehab failed, but I felt you needed surgery all along."

When surgery is needed, orthopedic surgeons do excel. While surgery should be used only as a last resort—the pinnacle of the pyramid of care—it can be quite beneficial in some cases, particularly when normal movement must be restored to body parts. But keep in mind that the success of a surgical treatment is never guaranteed, even when performed by an experienced surgeon.

Osteopaths: These doctors use medicine, surgery, and other traditional medical approaches, along with chiropractic-like adjustments, to facilitate the healing process. Many osteopaths specialize in performing certain procedures. Some may focus entirely on surgery, for example, while others decide not to do spinal adjustments at all. How sad! It may be difficult to find one who does it all, but well worth the effort.

Podiatrists: Podiatrists are doctors who specialize in the treatment of injury or pain in the feet and legs. They can provide orthopedic, medical, and surgical solutions to problems. Unfortunately, many podiatrists have become more involved with foot surgery than with rehabilitation methods, such as foot orthotics and exercise programs. But many still exist who are highly skilled at providing non-surgical foot rehabilitation.

Dentists: Some dentists specialize in healing various injuries by working with the temperomandibular joint (TMJ) in the jaw. While it may be difficult to believe, a misaligned TMJ can have an impact on the body structure. The dentist will correct this problem—or help to prevent an injury in the first place—by making a mouthpiece for you that realigns the TMJ. This can make an enormous difference in the alleviation of body pain.

Clinical Ecologists: These healers, who are typically medical doctors, recognize that the food we eat and the compounds that we inhale and ingest can weaken body systems. Weak adrenal glands, for example, often are linked with chronic injury. The clinical ecologist will identify the allergens to which you are sensitive and the body systems that are affected. He or she then uses a variety of approaches to helping the body heal. The treatment may include nutritional guidance, vitamin/mineral and glandular supplements, environmental counseling, and chelation therapy for the removal of toxic metals from the body and fatty plaque from the blood vessels.

In addition to the therapies described above, the following treatments can be used individually or in some combination to heal injuries and pain:

Acupuncture: This Chinese therapy is based on the concept that certain body parts and organs receive a diminished energy flow if various points in the body become "blocked." The blockage can be caused by an injury or even by poor body movements during daily activities, such as lifting something heavy off the floor improperly. In either case, it will produce the symptoms of illness. Acupuncturists use tiny needles to "unblock" the points and traditional Chinese herbal medicine to promote healing. When performed by a highly skilled practitioner, acupuncture offers a wonderful and relatively safe way to heal many painful problems, especially when used in conjunction with body rebalancing.

Alexander Technique: This is an excellent method of training your body to move in an ideal way. It can enhance both athletic performance and everyday activities. Teachers of the technique will show you how to achieve body posture and movement that ultimately allow you to "self-adjust" the spine and pelvis, thereby avoiding the cost of having a professional do the job. The technique can help to relieve muscle tension and injury-induced spasms. It allows a chronic injury to heal and serves as a preventive measure against potential injury.

Applied Kinesiology: Via this technique, developed by chiropractor Dr. George Goodhart, the healer will test muscle strengths and weaknesses and then realign the spine and body by applying gentle touches to the head and body. In the hands of a sensitive and competent practitioner, applied kinesiology can help people of all ages to correct the musculoskeletal imbalances that cause injury or slow the healing process.

Autogenic Training: With this technique, you learn to relax your muscles and body through various types of meditation.

The therapy will reduce and control the muscle spasms that cause most injury pain, raise your "pain threshold" (the point at which you first feel pain), and destress your body to help prevent future injuries.

Biofeedback Training: A machine monitors your muscle tension and reinforces the progress that you make in relaxing the muscles as you practice a relaxation technique. As a result, you may be able to control the muscle tension and stiffness accompanying an injury, lessen pain, and heal more quickly.

Brain Synchronizers: These computerized machines "talk" to your brain through the frequencies of flashing lights and sound (transmitted via special sunglasses and stereo headphones). Much like other meditation techniques, this method will stimulate your brainwaves to promote relaxation. In doing so, it can stop muscle spasms, prompt healing, and prevent muscle and tendon injuries. The technique has two important factors working in its favor: It does not require any kind of training on your part, and it works immediately. One good brain synchronizer, in particular, is made by Inner-Quest of Little Rock, Arkansas.

Color Therapy: Certain colors (such as those in lights) are believed to aid the healing process. While color therapy can be used to enhance other methods, it may be hard to find a healer who practices the technique. *Color and Personality* (Samuel Weiser, 1952), a wonderful book by Dr. Audrey Kargere, can be used as a guide to color therapy.

Cranial Therapy: This treatment, practiced primarily by osteopaths and chiropractors, uses manipulation of points on the skull to realign the body structure and affect the body in a way that's similar to applied kinesiology. Although it may take a number of visits to achieve significant results, cranial therapy provides a painless, safe, and effective way to prevent and heal injuries.

Diathermy: This healing machine applies a high-frequency electric current to body tissues to increase heat. The process opens up local circulation and helps push through congested body fluids (edema or swelling) in the injured area to induce healing.

The therapy, which is performed under a doctor's direction, can be used safely on a daily basis. The doctor can determine if you have any particular problems that may make the therapy unsafe.

Electrical Muscle Stimulation: With this therapy, a direct or alternating current is used to break up muscle spasms. The therapy fatigues the muscle by making it contract repeatedly. As a result, the spasms stop, the muscles relax, and the pain is relieved.

Galvanic Electric Therapy: This therapy is applied by a machine that uses a galvanic electric current to stimulate muscles safely and cause them to contract. The treatment can be very beneficial in helping to break up muscle spasms. In addition, it may facilitate the transmission of various medications through the skin and to the injured area.

Heat Therapy: This group includes hot moist packs, hot towels, hot clay, hot baths, hot air, saunas, paraffin baths, and similar treatments. All of these methods can do an effective job of stimulating blood flow to the affected area. Heat therapy should not be used immediately following injury when the pain is severe. Allow forty-eight hours to pass before starting these treatments. If heat makes an injury feel worse, use ice instead.

Homeopathy: Homeopathy focuses on the use of various safe substances such as arnica (an herb) to rebalance the body and promote healing. Homeopathic methods can be beneficial if they are used soon after an injury takes place.

Hydrotherapy: With this therapy, hot water (and sometimes cold) is used to increase circulation to the injured area and lessen muscle spasms. This will alleviate pain and induce healing, provided that the therapy is used forty-eight hours or more after the injury takes place. The water can be applied through whirlpools, hot tubs, and hot baths.

Hypnotherapy: Through hypnosis, you can achieve a trance-like state of mind that allows you to relax muscle spasms. The effects of the therapy are similar to those achieved with various forms of meditation.

Ice Therapy: Ice should be applied immediately following any type of injury. The best approach is to alternate ten minutes with the ice on the injury and ten minutes with it off as much as possible during the first twenty-four to forty-eight hours. A ten-minute ice massage to an injured bone or muscle often will completely numb it. The next step is to get an accurate diagnosis of the nature of the injury from the appropriate type of doctor, such as a podiatrist for a foot injury.

To make a safe and effective ice pack at home, fill a plastic, sealable food bag with enough ice to slightly surround the injured area. If the ice pack is too cold, wrap some paper towels around it. Avoid the use of synthetic ice because it may freeze the skin to lower temperatures than does regular ice. People with poor circulation and circulatory diseases must be especially careful when using ice therapy, even if the ice is natural rather than synthetic.

With some injuries, you may not know whether to use ice or some form of heat, such as hot baths and whirlpools. When in doubt, the safest strategy is to use ice therapy. In addition, any time you use a heat treatment and the pain or discomfort feels worse rather than better, switch to ice.

Magnetism: With this therapy, negative-pole magnets are applied to the injured area. Electrical bone stimulators or electromagnetic machines may be used as well. Depending on the method used, the therapy can reduce swelling or cause calcium and other minerals to reenter and heal the bone and muscle tissue. Magnetism offers an excellent way to heal an injury quickly.

Massage: The many schools of massage include Swedish, Myotherapy, Rolfing, Neuromuscular, Acupressure, Tragerwork, Shiatsu, Amna, Reiki, and others. With all of these techniques, the muscles, soft tissues, and energy points are pressed, rubbed, pinched, stroked, kneaded, and tapped to stimulate healing, break muscle spasms, and enhance circulation. Massage also helps the body to release endorphines and other chemicals naturally that control pain and release blocked energy. The various types of massage can do a fine job of speeding the healing process.

Physical Therapy: Physical therapy encompasses the use of exercise, massage, and various healing modalities (such as a whirlpool) to treat injuries that affect the bones, muscles, tendons, and ligaments. These techniques, which are practiced by licensed and trained therapists, can help the specific injury to heal and the rest of the body to rebalance.

Polarity Therapy: This method combines the light pressure of massage with a stretching and nutrition program to rebalance the body following an injury. When used in conjunction with other treatments, polarity therapy is a good way to help control pain and stimulate healing.

Ultrasound Therapy: The ultrasound technique creates heat with the use of high-frequency sound waves. This promotes circulation and breaks up any abnormal calcifications of bone and muscle, as well as pockets of swelling. It should not be used by elderly people, growing children, or anyone with severe osteoporosis.

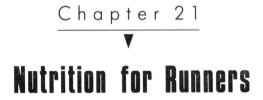

Chapter 21
▼

Nutrition for Runners

Nutrition plays a crucial role in a runner's overall health and performance. Training creates stress on the body systems and depletes the fuel supplied by food. Therefore, these nutrients must be replaced in a way that meets your body's individual needs. By developing a customized nutrition program, you can accomplish this goal and accommodate the specifics of your exercising regimen as well.

The following dietary issues, which are discussed in greater detail in the section on nutrition, must be considered by runners when they begin an exercise program. These nutritional issues include everything from the impact of food allergies on the body to the proper way to eat before and after exercising.

Allergies

Because allergies can have a tremendous impact on a person's energy level, runners must determine if they are allergic to any foods. An allergy can impair the functioning of the immune system. This, in turn, makes you more susceptible to infections, viruses, and other invaders. In addition, aerobic training typically causes some inflammation in the body, and a strong immune system is needed to facilitate the healing process.

Fats and Protein

When you begin an exercise program, make sure that you are getting enough fatty acids because the body will utilize a higher than normal percentage of fats. Such foods as raw seeds and nuts, grains, and avocado contain unrefined oils, the best and most natural source. Extra oil can be obtained from vegetable-based oil products. Avoid eating animal fats and the refined oils found in such foods as french fries and cake because you may consume a large quantity of unstable molecules. These molecules, called "free radicals," can attack cells and sap your body's strength.

Modify your consumption of protein, which takes a long time to digest. Complex carbohydrates are a much better choice for resupplying the body with glycogen, the fuel that provides energy. Protein, for its part, is an inefficient fuel that begins to serve the body only after other sources have been depleted. It uses a lot of body water in the digestion and elimination processes, increasing your chances of becoming dehydrated. When you do eat protein, stick with small servings. Your body can only digest and utilize three ounces of protein at a time. To eat a large serving would simply waste valuable energy.

Carbohydrates

On days when you perform aerobic exercise or compete in a short-distance race, eat a moderate amount of complex carbohydrates up to five hours beforehand to replenish glycogen. (Diabetics and people who have eating disorders should eat two and one-half hours before exercising.) In addition, be sure to eat enough so that you will not become hungry during the exercise period or the race. Avoid fat and protein, simple sugars, and spicy or salty foods. And allow time for the stomach and small intestine to empty before you begin.

Until one hour before the event, drink water or very diluted fruit juices. At that point, continue to drink water only. Surprisingly, you may not need to urinate during the event despite the consumption of fluids. When you are exercising, the functioning of the kidneys slows, and the body retains fluids that other tissues will use to promote sweating and lower body heat. In essence, the body's retaining mechanism overrides the eliminating system.

When preparing for a long-distance event such as a marathon, many runners practice a nutrition regimen called "carbohydrate loading." The eating plan typically works as follows: Seven days before the competition, the runner engages in a heavy workout that uses up any stored glycogen (carbohydrates) in the body. He or she also depletes the glycogen level by eating food that's high in protein but low in carbohydrates and fat.

Three days before the event, the diet is switched. The runner eats large amounts of carbohydrates to rebuild the glycogen level and keeps his or her protein and fat intake to a minimum. Because the body was deprived of carbohydrate fuel in the previous days, it should respond to the stress by delivering extra glycogen to the muscles, where it is stored. This process may provide the runner with more energy and allow him or her to go longer distances without tiring.

Two variations of this carbohydrate-loading technique exist: The first modification is to taper off the exercise schedule and rest during the week prior to the event, rather than to overwork the body with a heavy workout. The runner eats a high complex carbohydrate diet during the last week. The second variation also calls for rest and a high complex carbohydrate diet for forty-eight to seventy-two hours preceding the event.

Supplements

Some people cannot absorb all the vitamins and minerals contained in the foods that they eat, generally due to such problems as chemical imbalances, improper food combining, and sensitivities to certain foods. These people may need larger doses of supplements to compensate for a deficiency or to bolster certain inherent weaknesses.

People who exercise regularly—and stress their body in the process—may need the following supplements: Vitamin A to activate the immune system; B-Complex vitamins to replace those lost due to stress; Vitamins C and E and selenium to serve as anti-oxidants; and a one-to-one blend of magnesium and calcium to benefit the muscles. All athletes, and particularly women, should be tested for an iron deficiency before they start an exercise program and at least once or twice a year thereafter.

Eating at Night

If you eat a large meal in the early evening, you will hinder the natural process of recovery that takes place in the body at that time of day. It's a better idea to make dinner the smallest meal of the day. In addition, stop eating at least one hour before you go to bed. Anything you eat will take that long to digest, and whatever is in your stomach when you lie down will remain there and put added stress on the body. If you must eat late at night, stick to something light, such as a piece of fruit or such liquids as herbal teas or fresh vegetable juices.

Post-Exercise Nutrition

The water lost during exercising needs to be replaced as soon as possible to rehydrate the body and to lessen the fatigue caused by exercising. Eating can come later, after the body has had a chance to return to its pre-exercise functioning.

When you finish your exercise routine, drink 8 to 10 ounces of water immediately and every 20 minutes thereafter during the first hour. It doesn't pay to gulp down several large glasses at once. The body will only eliminate what it cannot absorb. Following that, drink 8 to 10 ounces each hour. Don't worry that you're drinking too much. Healthy adults who work out consume an average of eight 8- to 10-ounce glasses per day.

Your post-exercise diet should include protein as well as carbohydrates to help repair muscles and other tissues. If you are starving when you finish your workout, you probably ran out of fuel because your glycogen supply was depleted. The body is now eager to begin rebuilding its fuel levels. In that case, your pre-exercise diet may need to be adjusted to include more complex carbohydrates.

Finally, do not take salt after exercising. Contrary to popular belief, the body loses very little salt when you perspire. The loss of water, in fact, leaves large amounts of salt behind. For that reason, salt pills should not be taken.

Chapter 22

▼

Equipment

It's easy to overlook the importance of good equipment when starting a running program. Shoes and clothing—the "equipment" of running—are not exactly complicated items, after all. Nonetheless, you should give some consideration to what you will wear when you perform any aerobic exercise, especially one that puts a great deal of stress on the feet, legs, and body.

Running Shoes

Choose good-quality shoes that offer sufficient protection for your feet and body. Cheap running shoes most definitely will not do the job, but expensive shoes may offer more features than you need. To start, look for a pair of shoes in the mid-price range that suit your particular needs.

A strong and powerful runner, for example, will need shoes that bend under substantial amounts of pressure. A thinner athlete with a lighter stride would do better with a more flexible shoe. Runners who are overweight or who strike the ground heavily should get shoes with a shock-absorbant mid-sole and a strong counter, the part of the shoe near the heel that stabilizes the foot. All runners need shoes with the proper width and sufficient toe room to prevent rubbing and other irritations.

If you have rigid or hypermobile feet, avoid shoes with a C-shaped lasting. The last, or the basic form of the shoe, can be determined by the shape of the soles. Those that curve inward like the letter C (or a reverse C on the right foot) can aggravate certain structural imperfections in the feet. Thus, straight-last shoes may be better for people with such problems. They also seem to be better for race-walking programs. Be sure to examine the various types of lacing systems to determine which will provide the most comfort for any imperfections in your feet.

Retire your shoes from running when the mid-sole section that provides shock absorbancy begins to wear out. This usually happens every 750 miles of use, so be prepared to replace your shoes as often as needed. Don't spare the expense. Running shoes serve as the primary source of protection from the stress that travels through your feet and legs. The shoes can be used for walking if they are still in good condition, but do not use the same shoes for both walking and running. Save your running shoes—and the protection they afford—for the real work.

Clothing

Pay attention to the materials and fit of your running socks, your shorts, and any other clothing that you wear. If your socks become thin or worn out, they may create blisters or fail to help absorb the shock. When selecting socks, avoid nylon or synthetic materials that cause perspiration. Try wool or wool blends, which repel moisture away from the feet, or Thermax mixed with cotton or wool. Some specialized choices include socks made to cushion the heel and toe areas and those made of materials that are "guaranteed" to prevent blisters.

Many of today's running shorts are made of lightweight synthetic materials that do not irritate the body. Whatever materials you choose, make sure your shorts fit comfortably at the waist and thighs. Those with an elastic band or tie string are good choices. In addition, the new running suit materials available in most stores will help to prevent any hyperthermic or hypothermic reactions by allowing water vapor to escape. At the same time, they prevent water droplets (from rain or snow) from entering through the material.

In the winter, you may want to wear clothing made of new materials that establish an insular barrier next to your skin. This helps your outer garments to absorb perspiration and prevent it from collecting on the skin. The less moisture on your skin, the less quickly heat will escape from the body. Two brand names are Thermax and Capilene.

When running long distances in cold weather, wear a wool hat and perhaps a wool ski mask on your face to enclose some body heat. You should open or even remove some layers of your clothing, however, if needed during the run. Remember that mittens keep hands warmer than gloves. In the summer, you can wear a thin cotton hat to shade your head from the sun and prevent heat reactions.

The Use of Weights

It's best not to use weights on your hands or ankles when you are running. Ankle weights, in particular, can add to the risk of injury by putting additional stress on the foot as it strikes the ground. In addition, lugging around extra weight while running is not the best way to strengthen your arms and legs. Alternative exercises for that purpose are discussed in Chapter 26. If you are determined to use hand weights, of course, be sure to choose lightweight ones.

Chapter 23
▼

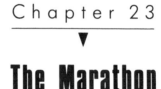

The Marathon

Marathon training is a long-term, intensive process of building up your endurance and acclimating the body to longer and longer distances. It will take a good eight months of diligent work to achieve the mileage and pacing needed to complete a 26-mile marathon. Don't be fooled by the training routines of top marathon runners, who knock out anywhere from 110 to 150 miles per week. They are professionals who have been training for a long time to reach that level of performance. The average athlete could seriously damage his or her body with that type of regimen.

Training

What follows is a suggested training program for a 26-mile race. By using this plan as a guideline, you can make the necessary adjustments to accommodate your schedule yet train properly for the strenuous event.

Month 1: Run 3 miles, 5 days per week.

Month 2: Run 4 miles, 4 days per week; run 8 miles on Sunday.
(Note: Tuesday, Wednesday, Thursday, and Friday would be best for the weekday runs. You could then rest on Saturday before the longer run on Sunday.)

Month 3: Run 5 miles, 4 days per week; run 10 miles on Sunday.

Month 4: Run 6 miles, 4 days per week; run 12 miles on Sunday.

Month 5: Run 6 miles, 4 days per week; run 14 miles on Sunday.

Month 6: Run 6 miles, 4 days per week; run 18 miles on Sunday.

Month 7: Run 6 miles, 4 days per week; run 22 miles on Sunday.

Month 8: Run 6 miles, 4 days per week; run 24 miles on Sunday.

At this point, you will be running a total of 48 miles per week—24 during the week and 24 on Sunday. In addition, you will have three solid months behind you of completing one long-distance run each week. If you do "interval training" on one of the weekdays, the training program will give you both endurance and speed.

Although it's important to build up your mileage, it's also essential to get plenty of rest during the training period. The weekday schedule above, for instance, could be modified to allow three days of rest instead of two. The long run on Sunday would stay the same, but the weekday mileage would be distributed unevenly among three days: 4 miles on Tuesday; 8 miles on Wednesday; and 10 miles on Friday. Monday, Thursday, and Saturday would be days off from running.

It's also important to alternate between short, fast-paced training sessions and ones that are longer and slower paced. If on some days you run 6 miles at a fast pace, switch to running 10 miles at a slower pace on other days. Finally, keep a daily diary throughout the training program to track the many factors (such as biorhythms and circadian rhythms) that influence your performance. This diary will help you to recognize the hidden cycles in your physical, emotional, and mental conditioning.

Pacing

Completing a long-distance race requires consistent pacing that does not stress the body. If you do shift pace in the course of a long run, the change must be methodical and it must progress from a slower pace to a faster pace. If you start out too fast, you'll be forced to slow down due to the buildup of lactic acid that the sudden, fast pace produces. As your body gets tighter and tighter, you will run slower and slower and may even be forced to stop completely.

A safer and more efficient approach is to start out slow and then increase your pace every six miles. Use a stopwatch to track your time for every mile. This type of pacing technique will keep you feeling good throughout the run. Since the body takes at least twenty minutes to loosen up, run at a warm-up pace for the first two miles. You may feel terrible during this time, but by the sixth mile you'll probably start to feel better. By the twelfth mile, you'll probably feel great.

To plan your pacing for a marathon, start by monitoring your time during the training sessions to determine your normal training pace. Then use that number to map out the pacing you want to achieve for each six-mile segment of the race.

Consider this example: During everyday training, a runner

determines that he can do twenty miles at an eight-minute pace per mile. In that case, he would start the marathon at a slower-than-normal pace to allow for some systematic shifts to a faster pace every six miles. His pacing plan would be developed as follows:

First 6 miles: 8:30 pace

Second 6 miles: 8:00 pace

Third 6 miles: 7:45 pace

Fourth 6 miles: 7:30 pace

At this point, he has reached the 24-mile mark and his *average pace* for the race is eight minutes, just as it is during his normal training sessions. With two miles remaining, he can either quicken or slow his pace, depending on how he feels. If he's still holding his pace easily, for example, he could run one more mile at an even pace and then put all of his energy into running at a faster pace during the last mile.

In any event, completing a marathon is no easy task. You could arrive at the 23-mile mark feeling that you still have plenty of energy and then come to an abrupt stop. Like thousands of others in the race, you have simply run out of steam. You can barely walk the last three miles, let alone run them. In most cases, this scenario happens when the runner has not properly prepared for the race in some major area—the pacing of his training was wrong, he trained too strenuously at the start, he didn't eat properly, or he peaked weeks before the run took place.

Many runners, in fact, will do poorly in a race because they are either overtrained or undertrained. When you feel your best during the training period, it may be time to ease up and rest for a few days so that you don't overtrain and begin to run on the downside of your peak. If you reach that state, you could be at greater risk for injury because the body is weak and therefore slower to heal. Your running form and foot placement could be off as well, setting you up for an injury.

When you finish the race, continue jogging for about twelve

minutes to avoid an abrupt stop. Then shift the pace from jogging to a brisk walk. Never, under any circumstances, apply heat to the body after the race. No hot showers, no hot tubs, no saunas.

Water

Drink at least one pint of water before the marathon begins. Then, throughout the race, drink some water every mile. The best way to consume water while you run is to sip it from a plastic container. If you can't have someone meet you at every mile with another container, however, this will not be possible. If you do drink from a cup, be careful not to gulp the water down. You could get stitches (intestinal cramps) if you gulp air as well. Although belching will relieve the stitches, many people cannot learn to belch. They may want to take charcoal capsules, which absorb any gas molecules in the stomach and intestines.

To delay your body's need to dip into its glycogen reserves, you can add some grape juice to your water. The grape juice provides extra glucose during the run, which helps to maintain your energy level without depleting your reserves. It's not a good idea, however, to take Vitamin C during the race because this vitamin often serves as a laxative. Finally, put an ice cube in your mouth if you feel nauseous during the run. It may help to alleviate the feeling.

Form

Good form is essential during a long-distance run. It will affect your energy level, the way that your body feels, and the amount of oxygen that you receive. To start, hold your head high and keep your shoulders loose. Your hands should swing lightly, with the wrists held at about hip level. You could cause muscle contractions if you position your arms any higher. In addition, any muscle fatigue in the shoulders will cause your arms to raise and your shoulders to slump. Consequently, you get less air and less oxygen is supplied to the cells.

Now, the lower body. Keep your feet as close to the ground as possible when you run. Bend your body forward at the waist just slightly. Do not run in a stiff-legged manner, which tends to jar the knees. Your knees should be slightly bent. When you run uphill, adjust your posture and form accordingly. Raise your elbows a bit behind you, shorten your stride, and run more toward the ball of the foot. Your knees should still be bent. When coming down the hill, put your shoulders forward to use the momentum.

Gear

Check the condition of your shoes before the marathon and break in a new pair if necessary. The old pair should not be used if the insole is flat and no longer provides any cushioning. An even more obvious sign are run-down heels, which can alter the body structure and lead to tendinitis, strains, and hip problems. In addition, you may want to have the curved pieces of leather on the backs of your shoes cut off if they irritate your feet during long runs. These tabs can rub against your feet throughout the run and may bruise the Achilles tendon. Wear thin socks that fit snugly and are in excellent condition.

In the summer, wear clothing that allows you to perspire properly. Even in the winter, do not overdress. Perspiration that cannot escape from your clothing could cause you to have severe chills in cold weather.

Before the race, take the following steps: Clip your toenails to prevent them from cutting into your toes. Put petroleum jelly around your heels, the balls of your feet, and all of your toes. Use it on your groin area, your breasts, and your armpits as well. Pack a small plastic bag (to be carried on you during the run) with electrolite tablets, charcoal capsules, and some tissues to wipe sweat from your face and even to use as toilet paper.

The following diet should be followed the week before the marathon: Eat protein only three times a day, on the fourth, fifth, and sixth days before the run. High-quality sources of protein include protein powder, soybean powder, and tofu; do not eat animal fat. You can have salads and beverages, but no grains, cereals, or fruits.

Three days before the race, drop the protein and switch to complex carbohydrates only. The day before the race, eliminate all fruits and salads. Eat something that will clear your intestines before the race begins. At about eleven o'clock that night, an hour or so before you go to bed, have a large meal that will pack your body with glycogen. Buckwheat pasta, whole-grain pasta, brown rice, and whole-grain bread are some good choices (as long as you are not allergic to wheat, of course). Do not eat spicy, greasy, or sugary foods. Sugar, in particular, will prompt the pancreas to produce extra insulin. As a result, you will reduce your blood sugar level and remove stored glycogen from the liver and muscle cells.

On the morning of the race, blend two bananas with grape juice if the race is at *least* four hours off. The body will digest this before the race, and you'll have some extra carbohydrates. Do not eat any solid food. You're likely to be nervous and the body will not digest the food correctly. Take two electrolyte tablets before the race and one every five miles. When the race ends, take another two.

In addition to eating properly, you may want to float in an isolation tank several times before the race. The day before the run, in particular, is a good day to float. You may want to get a massage as well.

▼

Part Three

The Larger Picture

Chapter 24

▼

Types of Exercise

At any age, the definition of being "fit" must include some recognition of the role of regular exercise. Granted, the workout that's most appropriate for an individual's physical condition may change as he or she ages. But the fact that exercise can help us to understand the vital link between our bodies and our minds will remain constant all of our lives. With the six types of exercise described here, you can accomplish almost any fitness goal, from improving cardiovascular strength and other internal functions to reshaping the body and gaining physical strength.

Aerobics

By definition, aerobic exercises use major muscle groups in a rhythmic, continuous manner and use oxygen to create muscle energy and enhance its delivery throughout the body. Aerobic workouts lead to a greater lung capacity, a stronger heart, larger blood vessels, and more capillaries. These "training effects" help the heart to pump more blood to the capillaries, which, in turn, deliver the blood to muscles. Waste products, such as carbon dioxide, are then exhaled.

The roster of aerobic workouts proves that this type of exercise can be quite strenuous: Running, walking, swimming, cross-country skiing, and bicycling all make the list. While these exercises place stress on the body, they also improve the body's ability to handle stress by increasing the cardiovascular and circulatory system's capacity to utilize oxygen. Hence, a positive cycle is set in motion. The more aerobics you do, the better your body functions. It can then reach even higher levels of performance.

During an aerobic workout, the body receives the oxygen it needs to burn glycogen and free fatty acids, both of which are essential fuels that allow the body to function. The exercises also increase a person's stamina and strengthen muscles by using the major muscle groups in a repetitive and rhythmic fashion.

To provide these benefits, the exercises must get your heartbeat into the target range (see Chapter 3) for 20 to 30 minutes, three to five times per week. When you run out of fuel, you can no longer perform the exercises. Hence, the target rate should not be exceeded. By overdoing it, you can deplete your supplies of fuel, run out of oxygen, and become too exhausted to continue. Then the benefits that you desire will be lost.

Anaerobics

Anaerobic exercises differ from aerobics because they are performed "without oxygen." The exercises typically use an intense burst of energy for a short time period, such as when you are running a 50-yard dash. The body's existing level of oxygen allows it to perform the short, explosive task, along with the energy produced by muscle cells that require no oxygen. If any more demands were to be made on the body, however, it would run out of steam quickly. Lactic acid builds up due to the muscle use, which is then converted to energy by a special process. This only works for seconds, however, not for minutes or hours.

Some classic types of anaerobics include weight training, sprinting, and golf. While these exercises may build strong and well-toned muscles (as opposed to the lean and flexible muscles produced by aerobics), the primary goal of your exercise program should be aerobic conditioning.

To improve specific muscle groups, you can either choose another type of aerobic exercise or use anaerobics to develop those particular muscles. In addition, many sports require good overall conditioning and the development of specific muscles, which means they qualify as both anaerobic and aerobic exercising. If you move continuously while playing tennis, for example, the exercise is aerobic. But the quick and intense energy that it takes to serve the ball is an anaerobic exercise.

Isometrics

These exercises involve no real movement; instead, they increase the size and strength of a particular muscle by pitting it equally against another muscle ("iso" for equal; "metric" for measure). To perform isometrics, you partially contract a muscle and then hold it in that position. This must be done with care, though. A sustained muscle contraction can cause the blood pressure to rise and the heart functioning to become irregular. In the worst-case scenario, this can cause a heart attack.

Isotonics

Isotonic exercises, meaning "equal tension," also increase the size and strength of specific muscles. Unlike isometrics, however, isotonics involve movement of joints while you are contracting a muscle, such as during weight training. They do very little for overall physical fitness or heart functioning. Even a well-muscled person can be in such bad shape that he or she has no endurance for even short-distance runs.

Isokinetics

These exercises involve constant motion and the application of force throughout the entire movement. An example would be to lift a weight and lower it with your own muscle power, rather than to lift it with your muscles and let gravity take it down as happens with isotonic exercises. With the Nautilus machine, for example, a muscle applies constant force throughout its range of motion. At points where the muscle reaches a partial resting position, the machine adds some "resistance" to force the muscle to exert energy.

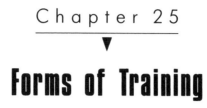

Chapter 25

▼

Forms of Training

People exercise for a wide variety of reasons, such as to improve their overall health and fitness, enhance their physical appearance, or acquire the skills and conditioning needed to participate in a sport. But whatever the specific goal, one rule about exercising always remain the same: To benefit the body in any substantive way, a training program must stress the body so that it will exceed its everyday performance. Even then, the exercise will only have a major impact on the muscles it puts to use.

Therefore, an effective training program must match the benefits sought by the athlete with the specific effects that a given type of exercise has on the body. In some cases, more than one form of training can be used to balance out the effects that each will provide. Once the desired level of fitness has been reached, the athlete then must maintain the beneficial effects.

The following forms of training can be used to achieve peak performance in different areas:

Aerobic Training

This type of endurance training derives its benefits from three crucial factors: the duration, intensity, and frequency of the workout. The proper duration of the exercise will depend on an athlete's conditioning and progress, while the frequency can vary from three to seven times per week. The intensity, as measured by the heart rate, must stay within the athlete's target range.

As a general rule, the "training effect" will come from 20 to 60 minutes of aerobic exercise at the target heart rate on three to five days per week. While the goal of aerobics is to improve cardiovascular endurance, remember that distance does not enter into the equation. The real results come from the combination of intensity and duration; the number of miles you run does not make a difference.

Interval Training

This combination of aerobic and anaerobic exercising improves both speed and endurance. The sequence works as follows: During the aerobic workout, you get close to your maximum heart rate for 30 to 60 seconds and then "rest" (ease up) for 30 seconds at about 70 percent of the maximum rate. Remember that if your heart rate drops below 60 percent during the "resting" period, the aerobic effects will be lost. Repeat the sequence three to five more times.

This training technique can be applied to any type of aerobic work, including running, walking, bicycling, and swimming. Once the body becomes accustomed to the method, you can make the training more demanding in the following ways: Increase the number of sequences, the intensity of the sprinting, or the length of the sprinting period. The length of the rest period could be reduced as well.

Fartlek Method

This technique is an informal variation of interval training. At different points during the aerobic workout, you simply speed up for a short distance or until you begin to feel the *first* signs of becoming "winded" or out of breath. Via the Fartlek (Swedish for "speed play") method, you do the training by feel rather than by timing your sprint with a stopwatch. Examples: sprinting up a hill, passing someone you see in front of you, or racing to the next light pole. The method can be used anywhere from four to ten times during the workout.

Circuit Training

This form of training includes a series of isokinetic and isotonic exercises that strengthen the muscles used in a particular sport. A coach or trainer identifies those muscles and then develops an exercise program aimed at building them. In most cases, the athlete will perform the exercises in a given time frame at various "stations" set up in the gym or on the field. The circuit is organized so that the athlete will not use the same muscle two times in a row.

The athlete's ability to maintain his or her target heart rate will determine the time limit for each circuit. If the heart rate exceeds 85 percent of the maximum, the number of repetitions should be decreased to prevent excessive stress; if the heart rate slips below 60 percent, however, more repetitions should be added. Aerobic exercise (such as riding a stationary bike) may be used in between stations.

Local Muscle Endurance and Strength Endurance Training

Local muscle training focuses on a particular muscle's ability to sustain a given level of work. It works at the cellular rather than the cardiovascular and circulatory levels. Your body's ability to use oxygen efficiently and remove metabolic wastes from the cells will determine your level of endurance. Wrestling and crew rowing, for example, require local muscle endurance as well as good cardiovascular conditioning.

Strength endurance training, on the other hand, helps you to put out a lot of muscle power over and over again without becoming fatigued. When a sport requires intense and repeated bursts of energy, as do basketball and football, the athlete needs both strength endurance and cardiovascular conditioning.

Chapter 26

▼

Alternative Exercise for Runners

When running does so much to improve physical conditioning, why would you need any other type of exercising? The answer is partly emotional and partly physical. On an emotional level, a change of pace can revitalize your approach to fitness by relieving any boredom with the regular exercise routine. On a physical level, other types of exercise can either support or supplement the benefits provided by your current regimen.

While running builds internal systems and leg power, for example, it has a limited effect on upper-body strength. Other types of aerobic work will balance muscular use and development while continuing to improve overall endurance. Anaerobic alternatives, on the other hand, will increase the strength, endurance, and skill of specific muscle groups. Finally, a regular or occasional break from running allows your legs to recover from any bouts of heavy stress.

Aerobic Alternatives

The ground rules for running apply to all other types of aerobic exercise as well. Do the exercise for 20 to 30 minutes three to five days per week. Perform the pre- and post-run routines with any aerobic workout. Start slowly with the alternative exercise and build your endurance gradually, adding about 10 percent every two weeks to the length of the aerobic work. Always use good-quality equipment.

Remember the basic rules for the post-exercise period as well. These include: Check your pulse immediately afterward to ensure that you reached your target range. Avoid anything that will restrict the flow of blood back to the heart, including weight training (do it before the aerobic workout, not after) and hot saunas, showers, and whirlpools. Be sure to rehydrate yourself to replace body fluids.

Cross-Country Skiing

This exercise may provide even more aerobic benefits than running, according to some experts. The sport requires you to use muscles in your upper and lower body, which increases the aerobic effect. You can ski outdoors during the season or use indoor cross-country skiing machines year-round.

Swimming

Swimming not only provides an excellent cardiovascular workout but also uses major muscle groups in a rhythmic manner. As a result, you can increase your flexibility while building more powerful arms, shoulders, and rear leg muscles. The pressure on bones and joints is minimized because of the water's buoyancy, which makes swimming ideal for people who are injured or those who have structural problems that prevent them from doing such aerobic work as running or bicycling.

Non-swimmers should start a swimming regimen by walking in the water. After taking your pulse, simply walk slowly from one side of the pool to the other in water that's about waist high. Build up the intensity of the workout until you have reached your target heart rate and can sustain it for 20 to 60 minutes.

Another technique to try is deep-water running, essentially a leg-intensive workout in which you "run" in the water while wearing a special life vest. Deep-water running can supplement a running program or help to heal an injury by building muscle strength. At first, you may only be able to sustain the motion for 1 or 2 minutes. But the goal is to work up to at least 30 minutes of continuous work. Any style of running can be used, with speed and range of motion as the variables.

People who know how to swim can develop a program that resembles the running routine—20 to 30 minutes of aerobic work on three to five days a week. In this case, do the pre-run routine described in Chapter 18 before you swim. Start with an easier stroke, such as the sidestroke or freestyle stroke, and gradually work up to your target heart rate. If necessary, swim on your back for a while to make it to the twenty-minute mark. Other people may be able to switch to a more demanding stroke, such as the butterfly or a breaststroke.

As with the running program, skip a day or two a week to allow muscles to recover from the stress of swimming. You can also use interval training with swimming to increase your speed and cardiovascular endurance. Sprint for up to 30 seconds and then return to your normal pace for 30 seconds. Repeat the sequence three to five times consecutively. When you finish swimming, be sure to stretch your rear leg muscles. If you used the backstroke, the anterior leg muscles will need to be stretched as well.

Swimming can only be your primary source of aerobic work if a pool is available year-round. If not, be sure to choose an alternate sport to complement the routine. In addition, try to find a pool where the water temperature is between 77 and 81 degrees Fahrenheit. Colder water makes it hard to warm up the muscles, while warmer water makes it difficult for body heat to dissipate.

Finally, protect yourself from ear infections and conjunctivitis of the eye by wearing a bathing cap (or ear plugs) and good-quality goggles that effectively guard the eyes. Do not, however, use a nose plug if your nose becomes irritated or inflamed. The water itself will do a better job of treating the condition. Watch out for any negative reactions to chlorine, especially if the pool contains high doses of the chemical. When swimming in the ocean, be prepared to use more energy to maneuver in the waves and currents.

Walking

The benefit of a walking routine is that it can be done just about anywhere, even indoors when necessary. It is also a more gentle form of cardiovascular exercise that people of all ages and all levels of physical conditioning can perform. It does take some time, however, to obtain cardiovascular results. It would take 90 minutes of walking, for example, to achieve the same aerobic benefits offered by a 30-minute stint of running.

The pre-run exercises should be used for a walking program as well. Be sure to take your pulse before you start. When you walk, use a rhythmic gait that takes the foot from heel to toe and allow your arms to swing naturally. Don't put them in your pockets or press them close to your sides. And try not to carry anything that will unbalance your body or add extra weight.

Walk 20 to 30 minutes on three to five days a week for the first couple of weeks. Every two or three weeks after that, increase the time by 10 percent until you have reached 90 minutes. Each time you walk, gradually build up to your target heart rate and then hold your pace. Check your pulse every 10 minutes or so. Slow down or stop if you feel tired, then slowly rebuild your pace.

The best walking surface is soft grass or earth. You can also walk on the street, of course, and even indoors if your health is poor or the weather is bad. In this case, walk in the hallways of your apartment building or inside your house, weaving in and out of the rooms.

Bicycling

This exercise provides a good complement to running because it affects a different set of leg muscles. While running primarily builds the rear leg muscles, bicycle riding will strengthen the anterior muscles in the front of the legs, thereby helping to prevent injuries to the rear leg muscles and the knees. Bicycling also puts less stress on the joints and muscles than running. However, injuries from collisions and pain in the knees, calves, and hands must be avoided.

To get the best cardiovascular benefits from bike riding, you must develop a steady pace that puts your heart rate into the middle of your target range. The cardiovascular conditioning that you desire will take a long time to achieve if the pace is too slow. A fast, sprinting pace, on the other hand, will lessen the training effect. Therefore, don't ride so hard that you continuously exceed 80 percent of your maximum rate. Use interval training to improve speed and stamina. Sprint for thirty seconds and then "rest" (ride more slowly) at your normal rate for 30 seconds. Repeat the sequence three to five times in a row. When you're done, be sure to stretch the legs properly.

Before starting a bicycling program, take the necessary safety precautions. Good-quality biking shoes will provide the most protection from the force of pedaling. The second best choice is to wear good running or walking shoes. Be sure to use foot clips to keep your feet on the pedals. Use a bike that's right for your height and that has a good, solid frame. Women often ride men's bicycles because the bikes tend to be better constructed as the crossbar makes them more stable. At the correct seat height, your knee will be slightly bent when the pedal hits its lowest point. Pant clips or rubber bands will keep your pants from getting caught in the chain. If you ride after dark, wear light-colored clothing that can be seen and use a red light on the bike.

When riding indoors on a stationary bike, follow the same guidelines as for outdoor riding. You can alleviate strain on your lower back and improve your body alignment by straightening up the handlebars from the racing-style position. Don't slack off because you are riding indoors. If you're reading a magazine as you ride, for example, then you're not working hard enough to get the desired aerobic effects. Generally, a more advanced bike—one with a computerized counter, for instance—will keep your attention and lessen the inevitable boredom.

Jumping Rope

If losing weight is one of your fitness goals, then jumping rope or simply jumping in place will burn more calories per minute than many other aerobic exercises. It's a tough cardiovascular workout, however, so you must begin quite slowly and build your tolerance over time. If the workout is too strenuous at the start, it could also seriously harm your lower back and legs.

On the first day, a healthy athlete should jump for two to four minutes only. A heavier or older athlete should do even less. Begin by walking or running in place, picking up speed until your feet are coming off the ground at a fast pace. Be careful not to pound into the floor heavily; be as light-footed as possible. Now, jump on both feet at the same time for 10 to 30 seconds, with or without a rope. Then rest by walking or jogging in place for a few minutes until you can breathe easily again. Repeat the process until you have jumped for no more than 4 minutes. The total workout time should be 20 minutes for beginners.

Do not overstress the body by jumping every day. Every two weeks, boost your jumping time by 10 percent. Eventually, you will be jumping for 20 to 30 minutes per workout, using interval training if desired. The gradual increase in duration will allow your bones and muscles to adapt to the stress. Doing "too much too soon" with jumping could damage your lower back and calves and even lead to stress fractures of the leg and foot bones.

You can either buy a jump rope or make your own. Simply get a ⅜-inch piece of nylon rope that doubles the distance from your nipple to the floor and then add two 6-inch pieces of PVC ½-inch pipes as handles. It's not important to use bearings or digital counters. As with all aerobic exercises, your heart rate is the real barometer of the cardiovascular benefits.

One benefit of jumping is that it can be done almost anywhere—in a small yard, a garage, a basement, and even inside your house or apartment if the ceilings are high enough to allow the rope to clear. Jumping rope is also a good option for people who travel a lot. In fact, you don't even need the rope to perform your aerobic workout.

Miscellaneous Aerobics

You may want to consider the following aerobic alternatives as well: using a treadmill, rowing in a boat or on a machine, roller skating, using a minitrampoline (or rebound jogging), and aerobic dancing. While stair-stepping also is aerobic, beginners should avoid it because it can prove to be too strenuous on the heart and knees. Other sports, such as basketball, tennis, handball, squash, and racketball, can provide aerobic benefits as well.

Anaerobic Alternatives

Weight training, racket sports, and golf all require sudden bursts of energy at times and then a lower level of energy output. Thus, they combine elements of both anaerobic and aerobic workouts. As with all anaerobic sports, they will improve the strength, skill, and endurance of specific muscle groups.

Weight Training

Runners often use weight training to increase the strength and flexibility of muscles throughout their bodies. Since weak body parts can lead to injury, this strategy helps the athlete to perform more safely and efficiently during long-distance running.

Your weight-training program should not emphasize the development of big muscles. Focus on strength, flexibility, and range of motion so that you don't end up with tight muscles and a greater body weight that hampers your running style. To complement the effects of running, the weight training should emphasize the development of the arms, shoulders, and anterior leg muscles.

Structure your weight-training program so that the body has forty-eight hours to recover between sessions. Since lifting weights breaks down muscle tissue, that's how long it takes for the muscles to repair. In the beginning, you should do three sets of eight to twelve repetitions with weights that are easy to lift. You get the greatest results when the muscle is fatigued, however, so the last two repetitions should be more difficult. These final reps build muscle strength, while the earlier reps provide better toning.

Increase the weight by 2.5 to 10 pounds when you can perform the last two reps with ease. To achieve specific benefits, alter the amount of weight you lift and the number of repetitions. Heavier weights and fewer reps (eight to ten per set) will build muscle mass; more reps (twelve to fifteen) with lighter weights will enhance muscle tone and increase strength. You should do two to three sets per exercise.

The different types of weight systems—including free weights, universal machines, and Nautilus (or any isokinetic) machines—all lead to the same basic results. They increase the size of muscles by taking them to the point of fatigue. Free weights help to develop better coordination than the other systems, but they also pose the greatest risks because the weights can fall. Although free-weight training can be performed at home or at a gym, it is typically more time-consuming because you must adjust the weights for each exercise. As a result, it may take you longer to perform your workout.

Racket Sports

These sports offer aerobic effects when the muscles are used continuously and during long volleys. The athlete needs endurance to work the court and sudden energy to make the shots. With the number of indoor and outdoor courts available in most cities, these sports are highly accessible.

Get a good instructor at the start who can teach you the right techniques and guide you to good-quality equipment. Remember that a cheap racket will affect your control of the ball and your ease of learning. Also, try to play with people who are at a similar stage of development with their skills and endurance. A far better player may only create tension and keep you from progressing at your own pace.

Golf

As with the other anaerobic sports, golf involves short, intense amounts of energy with each shot and then longer periods of relative inactivity. The shots require focused concentration and neuromuscular coordination, while a fast-paced walk between holes will improve aerobic conditioning. Indeed, you should always walk the course rather than ride a golf cart.

An instructor can teach you the proper technique at the start so that your stance and swing do not have to be corrected later on, a much harder proposition. Try not to bring your personal or professional problems to the course. If you do, the enjoyable aspects of the experience may be lost. As a final note, remember to drink plenty of water when you golf to prevent dehydration in hot weather.

Chapter 27

▼

Exercise and Weight Management

Any discussion of weight management must begin with a simple statement: The many diets that crowd the market today simply do not work. These weight-reduction plans have covered every possible approach to controlling food consumption—counting calories, eating high-protein diets, fasting on water—and every possible theory about how we can change our "attitudes" toward food and fat. Yet if even a few of the popular diets really did the job, why would so many new ones keep chasing at their heels, claiming to accomplish what the others have not? Within this environment, our society continues to consider obesity a sickness, one that must be overcome by depriving our bodies, taking drugs, and even undergoing surgical treatment.

We've also heard a lot about the "numbers" of losing weight. This extremely rational viewpoint goes as follows: Because 3,500 kilocalories equal one pound of weight, we gain a pound every time we exceed our energy needs by that amount, and we lose a pound every time our intake falls short by 3,500 kilocalories. Unfortunately, this approach to weight control doesn't work for the simple reason that our bodies don't operate like machines. As evidence, simply consider the heavyset people you know who gain weight when they barely eat at all and the thin people you know who never gain a pound no matter how much they eat.

What all of these failed diets tell us is that we need to take a more holistic approach to the issue of weight management.

Through a better knowledge of body functioning, we can begin to treat the cause rather than the symptoms of various weight problems. Each person can then use his or her own natural mechanisms to achieve individual weight-management goals.

The Setpoint

To understand weight management, it helps to understand the evolution of the built-in weight mechanisms that human beings have. Of necessity, primitive humans had a survival mechanism that stored fat when they gorged on available food and then conserved energy when they starved. When food was not available, the mechanism slowed down the metabolism and used just enough energy to keep the body going.

That same mechanism continues to work in us today. The starvation message may be activated when we eat irregularly or reduce our calories. If so, the body will begin to conserve energy and store fat as a protective measure. It will store any food that it gets until it has reached a predetermined "setpoint," or level of fat, that the body considers necessary for its functioning.

In recent years, researchers have been studying this mechanism to determine how the body gains and retains weight. At the crux of the issue is the hypothalamus, which serves as a control center in the brain to regulate body weight. It is the hypothalamus that determines what "setpoint" it considers best for your body and then maintains that level of fat.

The setpoint works much like a thermostat, according to the authors of *How to Lower Your Fat Thermostat*, a book that sets forth the concepts of a weight-regulating mechanism and setpoint. Just as a thermostat set at 75 degrees will activate the furnace when the temperature falls below 75, a setpoint of 165 pounds will prompt the weight-regulating mechanism to store more fat when the body weight falls below 165.

One way the mechanism maintains the setpoint is to control a person's appetite. In essence, it makes you feel hungry by sending you a signal to eat. Granted, you can't do anything to stop these urges. You can, however, exercise total control over the way in which you respond to the urges. Remember that the hypothalamus will activate the feeding mechanism until your weight returns to the setpoint. But you are the one to decide which foods you will eat and in what quantity.

The weight-regulating mechanism also monitors the setpoint by telling the body whether to store energy or to expend it. The body decreases the rate at which calories are burned when you do not eat much food; it increases that rate when you eat a lot. Either way, the objective is to keep your body weight at the setpoint. Consider the type of people known as "repeat dieters." Many of these people successfully lose weight for a short period of time, only to return to the former weight that represents their setpoint. The body does what it must to maintain its safety level.

In addition, studies have shown that thin people eat more than fat people, confirming many overweight people's claims that they eat conservatively. Overweight people, it seems, store fat more efficiently than they burn it. Their body chemistry can make fat from a diet that's low in calories to preserve the setpoint. Obviously, people who don't gain weight have a low setpoint. Their bodies use energy efficiently and do not store fat.

Lean Body Mass

Rather than focus on the presence of fat and a person's ability to gain weight, we should look at that same person's *lack* of lean body mass, which inherently prevents weight gain. When a person gains weight, after all, the muscles have decreased in fiber size. The collapsed or empty fat cells in and around the muscles then fill with storage fat. The fat inside the muscle is known as intramuscular fat. The fat that deposits outside the muscles is "subcutaneous."

Keep in mind, of course, that everyone must have some fat in the body. For adult men, the average amount of body fat is 15 percent; for women, the average is 22 percent. Ideally, men should have 5 to 12 percent of body fat, and women should have 12 to 15 percent.

When subcutaneous fat forms, a person will notice that he

or she is gaining weight from the resulting bulges. But more important than the changing body shape are the changes taking place in the muscles. As the muscles slowly become fat deposits, they lose their ability to burn calories. The chemistry of any remaining muscle alters and begins to conserve energy. Thus, gaining weight becomes a negative cycle in which the more fat you store, the more efficient you become at storing new fat. The less fat you burn off, the less efficient you become at burning fat.

To increase lean body mass, intramuscular fat must be replaced by muscle. And that's where exercise enters the equation. Exercising increases the amount of muscle tissue. And when you have more muscles, you also have more enzymes within the muscles to burn calories while you are exercising. The relationship between muscles and calories thus becomes a positive one: When the muscle volume increases, the fat level decreases and the muscles' calorie-burning function improves. *Therefore, the way to increase lean body mass is to move your muscles—and that means exercising.*

Developing a "Fit Cycle"

Running and other types of aerobics can help you to create a cycle of being fit rather than fat. The foundation of this cycle is the link between your energy input, or the amount of food you consume, and your energy output, or the type and duration of exercises you perform. By developing the right relationship between these two elements, you can go a long way toward changing the natural setpoint of your body weight.

To lower the setpoint, you need to make aerobic exercise a regular part of your life. There is no quick and easy way to make such a fundamental adjustment. The same routine that benefits the body's cardiovascular functioning—twenty to sixty minutes of aerobics three or more times a week—also will alter the setpoint over time and allow you to lose weight.

It's the cumulative effect of exercising that counts, not the isolated gains of any one day's routine. Indeed, the body burns very few calories during the exercising period. But over time, the ongoing use of calories begins to change the body's chemistry. The lean muscle mass increases, creating more enzymes to burn fat, and the metabolic rate increases so that the body burns calories at a higher rate. This, in turn, will eventually lower the setpoint. Remember that the increased metabolic rate doesn't simply come to a stop when the exercise period ends. The body will continue to burn calories at a faster rate.

Clearly, this approach to weight management requires much more effort and commitment than taking a few pills or going on and off diets. But the payoff of regular exercise is more than worth the effort. Not only will you lower your setpoint, but you will also gain all the cardiovascular benefits of performing aerobic exercises. Your overall health will improve, giving you far more substantial gains than a lower body weight alone. And unlike "spot exercises" for the thighs or other body parts, which simply do not work, an aerobic workout will help you to lose weight all over your body.

If your primary fitness goal is to lose weight, all the pre- and post-run exercises contained in the Holistic Workout (Chapter 18) still apply. In addition to taking your pulse before you begin the program, record your body measurements. Don't be upset if you gain a few pounds after the first few weeks. Because muscle weighs more than fat, the weight gain shows that you are getting rid of intramuscular fat and gaining muscle volume. Also, a single-minded focus on pounds is a misguided approach to measuring improvements. The fit of your clothing and a tape measure will tell you what you need to know. Losing inches (typically in the very places that you had hoped to lose weight) means a lot more than losing pounds.

Eating Plans

The second major aspect of reprogramming your setpoint is to change your energy input; i.e., the amount of food that you eat. As stated earlier, the hypothalamus has control over the appetite mechanism; you have control over what foods you eat and in what quantity when responding to those hunger urges.

In general, most Americans should have less protein and fat

in their diets and more complex carbohydrates. Another safe bet for anyone interested in health: Eliminate all white sugar, white flour, and salt from your diet. Then cut out any foods that are processed, frozen, or canned.

The important step in controlling your response to hunger is to get in tune with your appetite thermostat. In many cases, people stop eating long before the body is satisfied or continue well past that point. If you consistently eat too little, you may prompt the "starvation message" in the body. As a result, the hunger urges will become all the stronger, eventually causing you to binge. If you consistently eat too much, on the other hand, you will become so stuffed that you disturb the setpoint. The chances are good that you will gain weight.

To satisfy the body's hunger urges and its satiety point, you should eat smaller meals more often, generally every four to six hours. With all of your meals, keep your intake of fat and sugar to a minimum. Remember that it's important to eat breakfast and a light lunch. Both should lessen hunger urges but not make you too full. A water-based soup with legumes, grains, or vegetables is high in complex carbohydrates and therefore a good choice for lunch. If you have a salad for lunch, make sure that the dressing is not loaded with fat and sugar. Eat some whole-grain bread as well so that you do not become hungry too soon. Have a small snack if you do get hungry before the next meal. You may want to eat until you are completely full during one meal, usually lunch. This will not only satisfy your natural eating drives but also get you through the evening without constant snacking.

By combining aerobic exercising with a good diet, you will establish a new setpoint and stabilize your body weight at that point. If you follow this dual regimen and still don't achieve the weight that you desire, however, you may have set a wishful but unrealistic goal for your body. If your body stabilizes at a higher weight than you wanted, the best approach is to feel good about yourself at that weight. Take heart in the fact that as long as you continue to exercise and eat sensibly, the new setpoint will hold. You won't have to jump from one new diet to another in an attempt to lose the same weight again and again.

Part Four

Nutrition

Chapter 28

▼

A Focus on the Basics

Many people would like to find a magical formula for proper nutrition, and unfortunately, the numerous food fads, nutrition myths, and oddball diets that are served up to the American public may appear to offer just that. Once the dust settles, however, we must return to the simple truth that "good" nutrition differs for each individual. Not only are we each biologically unique, but our own needs also change over time. The amount of nutrients a person requires may depend on his or her age, the strength or weakness of the immune system, his or her level of activity, and a host of other health and fitness factors.

In short, there are so many mitigating factors that determine our specific nutritional requirements that it's difficult to make broad statements about how to eat properly. Of course, we all need high-quality sources of the major nutrients, including carbohydrates, fats, proteins, vitamins, minerals, and water, to achieve optimal wellness. But the moment you begin to run or power walk, and especially when training for such endurance events as marathons, your need for certain nutrients will increase.

By consuming more caloric nutrients during long-distance training, you will prevent your body from burning lean muscle tissue *and* fats to generate the fuel it needs for long workouts. The longer, harder, and faster the workout, the greater the impact it will have on your individual "setpoint"—the internal thermometer that regulates your caloric expenditure and rate of metabolism. You can effectively change that setpoint so that your metabolism, even while you are sleeping, works faster and burns more calories and nutrients.

We also know that people need far more water when they are training in hot weather than when training in cold weather. Even under normal conditions, a person needs about eight ten-ounce glasses of water a day. Dehydration generally results from losing more water than you take in over a period of time—and failing to recognize symptoms such as weakness, dry skin, and infrequent urination. For that reason, long-distance athletes should take an impedance test at least every other month to determine their percentages of lean muscle tissue, fat, and water. The water content should stay at about 70 percent or slightly higher.

The quality proteins a runner needs can be obtained from vegetarian foods. Again, you will require a little more than usual when you are in training. An extra serving of grains or beans, for example, will provide additional proteins and fatty acids. Be sure to obtain at least 15 percent of your calories from fats. Runners can drop below that level because they burn a lot of fat, so they need to replace what's lost with unsaturated sources of fats.

In our experience, runners must get optimal amounts of such nutrients as Vitamins C, A, and B-Complex, as well as calcium, magnesium, zinc, manganese, and selenium, all of which contribute to overall health and a strong immune system. This can be done through a good-quality diet or through special supplements when necessary. Without these vital nutrients, a runner's immune system is likely to take a beating as the wear and tear on the body increases, mile by mile and week after week.

Runners should be aware that there are two completely different schools of thought regarding the use of supplements. Many nutrition-oriented physicians, chiropractors, podiatrists, and athletes believe that such nutrients as Vitamin C, dymethylglycine, and coenzyme Q10 play a key role in athletic performance. Members of the more traditional science and sports medicine community, on the other hand, suggest that they do not.

Rather than try to convince you of either side's merits, we believe that it behooves you to use common sense to determine whether you need additional nutrients. Many long-distance athletes are educated people in professional fields, and they can certainly use their own critical processes of evaluation and deduction to determine how their needs should be met. If you take extra Vitamin C, for example, and find that you have fewer infections, less muscle fatigue, and faster recoveries from strenuous workouts than when you don't take the supplement, then the experts' suggestions become irrelevant. Your own experience will be the path that you follow.

In reviewing much of the scientific literature available on this topic, it seems that many studies have given too little of a nutrient for too short a period of time to subjects with a poor dietary program. Some studies, for example, give a relatively small amount of an isolated nutrient to marathon runners who eat large amounts of sugar, refined carbohydrates, animal proteins, and dairy products. If the study concludes that the nutrient made no significant difference, perhaps it's because the project design was defective, not because nutrition plays no role in exercise.

By contrast, members of the Natural Living Running and Walking Club, a holistic club, eat a vegetarian diet, practice stress management, learn preventive exercising, stretching and relaxation techniques, and work under the guidance of sports doctors, podiatrists, chiropractors, holistic physicians, and top coaches, including Peter Roth, Dr. Howard Robins, Lou Calvonea, Dr. Alan Pressman, Dr. Martin Feldman, and Helene Britton. All of these experts recommend a holistic approach to exercising and nutrition.

In our careful reviews of these athletes' nutrient programs, we have controlled many factors in their diets by eliminating refined sugars, animal proteins, and common allergens and by monitoring their liquid intake. With this nutrition program as a base, the athletes will add a given nutrient in increasing amounts over a six-month period. This allows us to get a fairly accurate reading of whether that nutrient makes a difference as an athlete experiences highs and lows in his or her circadian rhythms, biorhythms, and recovery times. Based on the hundreds of runners who have participated in these reviews, we believe that such nutrients as barley grass, Vitamin C, calcium, magnesium, dymethylglycine, and others make a substantial difference.

While these results are meaningful, we still believe that athletes must focus first and foremost on the essential elements of a normal, healthy diet. Because the major nutrients can be obtained from many sources that vary significantly in quality, for example, athletes must learn to distinguish between the good and bad sources, such as complex versus refined carbohydrates, unsaturated versus saturated fats, and plant-based protein versus meat products.

In the chapters that follow, we lay out the fundamentals of good nutrition and guide you to the best sources of nutrients. We also tell you how to prepare these foods to facilitate digestion. Other chapters cover the role of vitamins and minerals, the impact that food allergies can have on your body, and the best approach to developing a supplementation program that will enhance your performance during marathon training.

Again, the best results from a change in diet will stem from a holistic approach to nutrition. Remember our friend who became a marathon runner and a vegetarian for all the wrong reasons. The lesson we learn from his experience is that good nutrition requires us to take a step back from specific goals—such as winning a race or losing weight—and examine the bigger picture. The primary purpose of eating properly is to become a person who functions well in all aspects of life, including the family environment, professional life, and the sports arena. When you maximize the fundamentals, you maximize the very way in which your body functions. Those who have special requirements—such as marathon runners—can then use this foundation as a launching point to modify their nutrition for specific events.

Chapter 29

▼

Digestion, Absorption, and Elimination

In some ways, it's nice to ignore the realities of what your body does with the food you eat, but when it comes to good digestion, ignorance is not bliss. By understanding the basic functioning of the digestive system, you'll also understand the role that proper nutrition plays in promoting health. Here we follow the process through its three principal stages: digestion, absorption, and elimination.

Digestion

The process begins as soon as you put food in your mouth. The teeth begin to cut and grind any food that is not already either liquid or mucoid in consistency. During this process, the food mixes with saliva to become a soft, mucoid mixture. Saliva, which is about 98 percent water, also contains ptyalin, an enzyme that begins the decomposition of starch into the simpler molecules of sugars and dextrins. Digestion is said to start in the mouth because of the presence of ptyalin. If a starchy food is chewed long enough, the sugar-rich substance will become sweet. This occurs when an enzyme called amylase breaks down the starch.

A person produces anywhere from three-fourths to a full liter of saliva a day, regardless of how much he or she chews. The saliva cleans and lubricates the mouth and tongue to prevent the inflammation that could be caused by friction against the teeth. At the sight, smell, or even thought of food, the amount of saliva increases as the mouth begins to "water."

Once the food has been reduced to a semi-liquid condition,

the tongue rolls it into a ball called a bolus. It then pushes the food back into the pharynx to be swallowed. Here the voluntary part of the digestive process ends and everything shifts into automatic. The uvula moves up to shut the nasal passages, the epiglottis covers the larynx, and the tongue prevents food from returning to the mouth.

At this point, the food can only move in one direction—down into the esophagus, a less than one-inch-wide canal behind the trachea that measures nine to ten inches long. The esophagus has muscle fibers that run both longitudinally and in ring-like circles. While the top few inches contain striated muscles, the bottom is smooth. In its lower depths, the esophagus passes through the diaphragm.

When the food enters the esophagus, it causes a dilation of the canal and a contraction of the longitudinal muscles. This, in turn, sets off a series of contractions in the rings of muscle that line the esophagus. Each muscle contracts as the food travels the length of the canal, thereby forcing it along to the next muscle. Because the food is still semi-solid, the muscular activity speeds up the process of transporting it to the stomach. (It also explains how people can swallow en while standing on their head.)

Just below the diaphragm, the last set of ring-like muscles typically remain contracted. These muscles are called the cardiac sphincter because of their close proximity to the heart, rather than to signify any cardiac functioning. As the food approaches, these muscles relax and the bolus enters the stomach, where it will generally stay for three or four hours before departing. As the largest section of the digestive tract, the stomach is the closest thing we have to a storehouse of food. In an adult, it has a capacity of up to 1.5 liters.

When hollow, the stomach is a J-shaped tube that presses against the diaphragm at the top. It is the broadest and most muscular section of the alimentary canal. The upper portion of the stomach, called the fundus, is usually inflated with a bit of gas even when the stomach is empty. The lower portion, or pyloris, serves as the gatekeeper of the stomach. The wall portion of the stomach contains longitudinal folds called rugae that flatten and disappear as the stomach fills with food. At this point, the stomach becomes pear-shaped. It can become especially distended in the upper portion when you are full. The lower part of the digestive tract also contains bacteria that are important for the decomposition of foods.

The sphincters at either end of the stomach remain contracted to enclose the food. The stomach then experiences peristaltic contractions that merge the food completely with the digestive juices it generates. The churning action of the food may produce "rumblings" due to the presence of gas in the stomach. When the stomach has been empty for a while, the peristaltic actions begin again and the rumblings may grow louder. The gas is compressed in the process and occupies a larger portion of the stomach volume. It then exerts pressure against the walls of the stomach and produces the sensation that we call "hunger pangs."

The stomach's inner lining contains up to 34 million small glands that secrete a stomach "juice." The highly acidic nature of this juice—it contains up to 0.5 percent hydrochloric acid—makes it an unusual body fluid. When the acidity is higher than usual, gas accumulates and increases the pressure against the walls, causing pain. To relieve that pressure, the gas must escape through the esophagus and mouth. On occasion, the gas bubbles carry some of the acidic juices up to the esophagus and produces the feeling of "heartburn."

If any major portion of food in the stomach has not yet become liquid, the pyloric sphincter between the stomach and the lower region of the alimentary canal remains closed. Eventually, however, the gastric digestion and juices reduce the food to an entirely fluid substance called chryme. At this point, the pyloric sphincter relaxes, and the fluid can pass into the next segments of the canal, aided by the peristaltic action. The stomach acidity has disposed of any bacteria originally contained in the food, making it nearly sterile for a short period of time. The bacteria will appear again in the lower sections of the stomach.

The chryme then enters the intestines, which are composed of two segments: the small intestine, which is actually the longest section ("small" refers to its width, not its length), and the large intestine. The entire length of the small intestine is required to make absorption reasonably complete. The duodenum, the first ten to twelve inches of the intestine, bears the brunt of the highly acidic chryme that flows through the pyloric sphincter. It neutralizes the acid with the mucus secretions that flow from two large glands.

The smaller of these two glands—but the second-largest gland in the body—is the pancreas. It measures about 6.5 inches long and lies along the back wall of the stomach, near the bottom of the organ. The pancreas is both an exocrine and an endocrine gland, meaning that it secretes both inwardly and outwardly. The pancreas's large main duct joins with the common bile duct at a sac within the wall of the duodenum.

The pancreatic juice flows into the duodenum through a duct located just below the pyloric sphincter. Some 0.7 liters of fluid pass through this duct every day, carrying with it a variety of enzymes that attack different types of foodstuff. These enzymes include a starch-splitting enzyme called the pancreatic amylase and a fat-splitting enzyme called the pancreatic lipase. The protein-splitting enzymes in the pancreatic sac include the pancreatic proteases and proteinases (formerly called trypsin and chymotrypsin).

Neither of the protein-splitting enzymes, which continue the work begun by pepsin in the stomach, can function in an acidic environment. Therefore, the acidity of the food released from the stomach must be neutralized by the pancreatic juices and by a solution created by the liver, the largest gland in the body and one of the most important "chemical factories." The liver, which weighs three to four pounds, lies over the stomach and to its right, just beneath the diaphragm. It consists of four lobes, with the extreme right lobe being the largest. The liver's primary function within the digestive system is to produce bile salts, which help to absorb the fats in the small intestine. It also serves as a warehouse of sugar, which is deposited in the form of glycogen.

The stomach chryme, now mixed with bile and pancreatic juice, travels from the duodenum into the main section of the small intestine, which consists of two parts called the jejunum and ileum. The small intestine is lined with villi, numerous little projections that give it a velvety appearance. The incessant movement of the villi facilitates the absorption process by keeping any solvents in the immediate area continually churning. The intestinal glands, a group of cells that lie at the base of every villus, secrete an intestinal juice called entericus into the canal. This intestinal fluid contains a number of enzymes that break down the elements produced by the preceding digestive processes.

Absorption

At this point, the job has neared the absorption stage. The intestinal fluid also contains enzymes called peptidases that break down the remaining protein fragments into amino acids, the fundamental protein building blocks.

Absorption through the intestines works much like absorption through the lungs. The elements of fat digestion enter lymph capillaries that are called lacteals because the droplets of fatty material change the lymph from opaque to milky. The villi's capillaries band into venules and then veins.

Finally, these veins unload into the portal vein (located just behind the pancreas), which transports the assimilated producers of amino acid and carbohydrate digestion to the liver. The portal vein then breaks up into sinusoids, a network of vessels throughout the liver that are somewhat broader than capillaries. Kupffer's cells, which exist along the walls of the sinusoids, act as scavengers by filtering out any debris in the blood, such as any bacteria that may have maneuvered the intestinal wall.

The cells rimming the sinusoids also divest the blood of its added supply of glucose and amino acids. The glucose is combined to form molecules of glycogen, a quasi-starch. Any galactose or fructose present is first converted to glucose and then to glycogen, which stays behind in the liver. The blood coming from the liver contains only a small, stable amount of glucose. It also has the proper amount of protein molecules because the amino acids are picked up by the liver cells in this form.

Once the blood in the sinusoids passes the liver, it is again collected into the hepatic vein, which enters into the vena cava (the body's largest vein) and, thereby, into the general circulation. The blood courses through the tissue capillaries, and the plasma trickles across the capillary borders and becomes intestinal fluid. As this process takes place, the various body cells assimilate the glucose delivered into the blood by the liver and break it down, preparing it for energy. They also assimilate the proteins, tear them apart, and construct their own particular varieties.

The liver will resort to its reserve supply of glycogen between meals, when the cells place a burden on the glucose supply that new glucose from the intestines does not instantly relieve. The glycogen, stored after a meal, is now reduced to glucose and fed slowly into the bloodstream. Within limits, the body can change one form of food into another. The liver, for example, can only store enough glycogen to get the body through about thirteen sedentary hours. If glucose continues to be satiated with glycogen, however, the glycogen must be converted from fat and stored in that form. Since fat is a more concentrated form of chemical potency than glycogen, it can be stored in definite portions. After a day or two of fasting, when the liver's supply of glycogen is drained, the body can utilize its fat storage as a reservoir of blood glucose.

Food takes about three hours to travel the distance of the small intestine and arrive at the gateway to the large intestine, the last significant section of the alimentary canal. The large intestine, called the colon, is about five feet long, and its major segment is divided into three sizable regions. The small intestine enters the large intestine near the groin on the right-hand side of the body. From this juncture, the first section of the large intestine, called the ascending colon, surges upward to the lower end of the ribcage. The next section, called the transverse colon, makes a swing to the left and passes under the liver, stomach, and pancreas. Finally, the descending colon heads downward again toward the left side of the hipbone.

The meeting point between the large and small intestines, called the ileocolic sphincter, is set about two inches above the bottom of the ascending colon. In essence, that means the part below that point forms a dead end. This section, the caecum, collects material and acts as a storage place where fermentation can occur. It can become swollen to the point that it constitutes half the total length of the large intestine and becomes a danger. The appendix, a four-inch long appendage at the bottom of the caecum, is the remnant from the time that it was a large and practical organ. The removal of the appendix (through an appendectomy) has become a relatively common operation in this century.

Elimination

The body uses a considerable amount of water for its many digestive secretions. The absorption of this water and other substances continues in the large intestine, where little actual digestion takes place. As the water is subtracted, the contents of the large intestine become increasingly solid. By the time the contents reach the lower section of the descending colon, they are solid but soft.

The large intestine makes an S-shaped curve at the lower end of the descending colon so that it can reach the middle of the hip region. This short segment is called the sigmoid colon. The last four to five inches of the colon, the rectum, are vertical. The anus is the opening at the end of the rectum that leads outside your body. It is closed off by the anal sphincter.

The solid contents, or feces, are composed of "roughage," which includes unassimilated residue of food, fragments of cellulose and similar substances, collagen, and other constituents of connective tissue. The bile pigments released by the liver give it a brown color. The feces also may contain bacteria, which can multiply rapidly in the large intestine. While most of the bacteria are not pathogenic, some can be extremely virulent. They include cholera, disentary, typhoid fever, and other such diseases that can be passed among people through the fecal contamination of water reservoirs.

Defecation, the act of eliminating the feces, results from the normal peristaltic activity of the rectum and the use of the diaphragm and abdominal muscles. This is generally preceded or accompanied by the release of intestinal gases referred to as flatus, which have an unpleasant fecal odor. The relatively harmless gas contains small amounts of vaporable compounds that are created by bacterial activity in the large intestine.

Chapter 30

▼

Carbohydrates

Over the years, carbohydrates have suffered from a bad reputation because many people identify them with fattening, calorie-laden foods. The crux of the problem is that low-quality carbohydrates, such as candy, soft drinks, and refined pastas and cereals, have been grouped indiscriminately with the healthy varieties, including whole grains, legumes, starchy vegetables, and fresh fruits. As a result, promoters of high-protein, high-fat diets have claimed that many people cannot tolerate carbohydrates, and doctors have warned their overweight, hypoglycemic, and diabetic patients off carbohydrates altogether.

Fortunately, carbohydrates have gained more stature in recent years as the health field got the word out that all carbohydrates are not created equal. While any carbohydrate-rich food will energize the body, the high-quality sources also offer essential nutrients that fuel the body in other important ways. When the right carbohydrates are eaten, in fact, they should account for roughly three-fourths of your total caloric intake.

The Need for Carbohydrates

Despite the misconceptions that surround carbohydrates, no one can deny that these nutrients are essential to our diet. They include starches and sugars, the storable fuels that supply us with the immediate energy we need to function, and nondigestible cellulose, the fibrous material that gives plants their shape.

Carbohydrates not only serve as our most important source of energy—currently supplying about half of our energy needs—but also play a crucial role in our metabolic functioning. Each gram of carbohydrate yields four calories of energy upon oxidation in the cells. Carbohydrate foods also provide us with vitamins, minerals, and amino acids. Indeed, they serve as the primary source of protein for people in many parts of the world.

Considering the importance of carbohydrates to our diet, athletes must learn to distinguish between the two basic types—the complex carbohydrates that have nutritional value and the empty starches and sugars that have lost their value through refinement. Unfortunately, this may be tough to do when some diets geared specifically at athletes imply themselves that one carbohydrate is just as good as another.

Endurance athletes who use "carbohydrate loading" techniques to prepare for a marathon, for example, could easily come across planned, pre-competition meals that recommend the following foods: pie, cake, cookies, sweetened fruits, coffee with sugar, iced tea with sugar, chocolate milk, cocoa, milkshakes, ice cream, and hamburger buns (which are likely to be refined). They would do much better, of course, to load up on complex carbohydrates than to put these empty calories into their bodies.

Complex Versus Refined

Complex carbohydrates are whole starches, sugars, and fibers in their natural state, having received little or no processing. The starches and sugars supply the body with energy, while the fibers help the digestive system to function properly and supply the body with protein and B-and C-Complex vitamins. The complex form of carbohydrates, which existed long before "refinement" came about, are best suited for our consumption.

Refined carbohydrates, on the other hand, have been stripped of just about everything that makes them nutritious—the outer shell, or bran layer, that contains most of the fiber, the natural oils, and the germ that's rich in Vitamin B. Refined flour, which contains no wheat germ, and refined cane sugar, which consists of chemically pure sucrose crystals, are mere shells of the complex carbohydrates that exist in nature. Thanks to the wonders of food processing, refined carbohydrates also may be bleached, milled, baked, puffed, or otherwise altered from their original state.

At the end of the production line, we get highly processed foods devoid of nutrients and fiber but loaded with pure starch and sugar. And the foods that dominate the production line have also come to dominate our diets, despite the fact that they can lead to poor intestinal health, various digestion problems, and blood-sugar disorders such as hypoglycemia and diabetes.

Consider the following foods that compose the typical American diet: Breakfast cereals, which are generally derived from wheat, corn, oats, or rice, rarely come in their natural form (with a few notable exceptions, such as real oatmeal and hot whole-wheat cereals). Instead, they are dried, refined, bleached, steamed, puffed, flaked, or sugared. While the producers sometimes "enrich" the cereals by adding back in some vitamins and minerals, the milk that people add to cereal provides most of the nutrients available from this meal.

Meanwhile, the breads we eat—including the "rye" and "whole wheat" varieties—feature refined flour and an abundance of chemical additives. The white rice that most Americans choose for its pristine appearance lacks the protein, fiber, vitamins, and minerals found in whole brown rice. And the potato chips that we snack on barely resemble the vitamin-and fiber-rich potatoes from which they are made.

Carbohydrate Requirements

Americans consume about half of their calories from carbohydrates, generally in a refined form. What we must begin to do is eliminate these processed foods from our diet and replace them with their complex counterparts. That means giving up candies, cookies, sugars, refined pastas, breads and cereals, and sugary beverages, including the sugar-loaded "fruit juices."

You can begin this process by recognizing the amount of carbohydrates found in various refined and natural foods. The percentages for refined products are as follows: bread, 55 percent; spaghetti and pasta, 75 percent; cereals, 80 percent; candies, jams, and other sugared products, 90 percent. The complex carbohydrates, by comparison, contain the following carbohydrate counts: green leafy vegetables, 8 percent; fresh fruit, 15 percent; starchy vegetables, such as corn and potatoes, 20 percent; dry legumes, 60 percent; and dry grains, 70 percent.

Ideally, complex carbohydrates should be the foundation of our diets, accounting for 75 to 80 percent of our caloric intake. Another 12 to 15 percent should come from complete protein sources such as animal meat, with the remaining 10 to 12 percent coming from the fats found in oils, nuts, and seeds. To achieve this optimum diet, we would have to obtain fewer of our calories from fats and complete proteins than we currently do. Our daily diets could then consist of three to four servings of fruits and vegetables and one to three servings of whole grains and legumes, preferably in a combined fashion so that the proteins in each source complement one another.

This diet is especially important for athletes. While fat serves as a backup source of energy in our bodies, carbohydrates (stored as simple sugars and starches) are the most easily converted form of energy. The sugar that we get from food may be converted into energy, starch, or fat by the body. We generally store about a thirteen-hour supply of glycogen (starch) and glucose (sugar). Our cardiac and skeletal muscles store about 225 grams of glycogen, and the liver stores about 100 grams. And our blood sugar level should maintain a steady circulation of about 15 grams of glucose.

Remember that the primary purpose of food is to supply energy. For that reason, a high-protein diet can be dangerous. As a building material, protein can be oxidized as a fuel, but the process of doing so is an inefficient way to supply energy to our body systems. It requires more energy and creates a waste product called urea that must pass through the kidneys to be eliminated. Therefore, burning protein as a fuel stresses and weakens the kidneys. Carbohydrates, by comparison, provide immediate energy. When they are oversupplied, the body simply builds up its glycogen reserves or converts the extra carbohydrates to fat.

Sources of Complex Carbohydrates

Consider the following food groups in adding more complex carbohydrates to your diet:

► *Grains:* This wide-ranging group includes whole wheat, rye, triticale (a cross between wheat and rye), corn, barley, brown rice, oats, millet, and buckwheat. Many people who are allergic to wheat can tolerate triticale. Grains can be served whole, as cereals, mixed in soups and casseroles, ground into whole flour, and baked as bread or rolled into whole-wheat pastas.

► *Legumes:* This category also offers a wide variety of complex carbohydrates. Common types of legumes include lentils, kidney beans, mung beans, split peas, black-eyed peas, soybeans and soy products, such as tofu, tempeh and miso, navy beans, red beans, pink beans, pinto beans, black beans, turtle beans, fava beans, chick peas (garbanzos), and peanuts.

► *Vegetables:* All vegetables contain carbohydrates. The starchier root vegetables, such as carrots, beets, potatoes, and yams, tend to be high in fiber and unrefined starches and sugars, while the lower-calorie varieties, such as celery, broccoli, and mushrooms, consist primarily of water and fiber.

► *Fruits:* These are an excellent source of natural sugar, fiber, and vitamins and minerals. While the sugar content of fruit is somewhat high, it will be released into your system relatively slowly as you chew and digest the pulp. As a result, your body won't get the sudden jolt from apples, oranges, peaches, and other fresh fruits that it does from refined, pure sugar. Bananas, other tropical fruits, and dried fruits such as figs, dates, raisins, and prunes contain even more sugar. The dried fruits, in particular, have three times more sugar than fresh fruit. They should be eaten only occasionally.

► *Seeds and nuts:* Sesame and sunflower seeds are high in protein and carbohydrates. Alfalfa, chia, and flax seeds (grown organically as food, not for use in fabric) are highly nutritious when sprouted. While most nuts consist primarily of fat, carbohydrates can be derived from almonds, cashews, pine nuts, and pistachios.

Preparing and Digesting Carbohydrate Foods

In recent years, a number of vegetarian cookbooks have been written that offer recipes for carbohydrate-rich foods from all nationalities. These should alleviate the fears of many people, and especially meat eaters, that a diet containing less protein and more complex carbohydrates will be dull.

Many delicious meals, in fact, can be created with carbohydrate foods. Seasoned grains such as millet can be stuffed into peppers, tomatoes, or zucchini. (You may want to mix the millet with soy granules or lentils to enhance the protein content.) Vegetables can be mixed with legumes to make stews, casseroles, and soups. And such seasonings as leeks, dill, oregano, and cumin can spice up the dishes without adding sodium.

When properly cooked, starchy foods such as beans and grains can be digested in sixty to ninety minutes, a relatively short amount of time when compared to proteins. Cooked starches are easier to digest than uncooked varieties because heat ruptures the cell walls of plants and allows the enzymes in the mouth and intestines to convert the starch to sugar more easily. The carbohydrates in fruits and fruit juices may be digested in about forty minutes.

You can speed up digestion by eating more fiber with your meals. The fiber will absorb water and stimulate the peristaltic action of the digestive tract, pushing the food along. Don't begin your meal with a beverage, however, and especially one that's cold. This will briefly dilute the acid in your stomach and slow down digestion. In addition, carbohydrate foods should not be eaten at the same time as animal proteins, which can take four or more hours to digest. If the carbohydrate foods also stay in the stomach during that time, the sugar may ferment in the warm environment and cause indigestion and gas.

Meals that require all four digestive processes—for meat, potatoes, vegetables or salad, and a dessert—will weaken your ability to digest each type of food. The acid for the meat protein neutralizes the amylase in your mouth and hinders the digestion of starch. The simple sugars from the dessert will begin to ferment and may cause a hyperacid reaction in the stomach. At this point, taking an antacid would disrupt the digestive process even more. Clearly, these eating habits could eventually cause chronic indigestion and stress on the gastrointestinal tract.

The best approach is to eat complex carbohydrates at one meal and protein at another, snacking on fruits in between. In fact, it's a good idea to eat a piece of fruit fifteen minutes or so before a protein meal. This will prevent your blood-glucose levels from slipping during the time-consuming process of digesting protein. This process depletes you of energy for several hours as blood from other parts of the body is supplied to the digestive organs. Indeed, if you eat protein at every meal, some portion of your energy may be diverted to the digestive process for the entire day. Therefore, it's a better idea to eat a few small meals that include complex carbohydrate foods. Most likely, your energy level will be higher and more consistent and your intestines will not be overstressed.

In some cases, people have trouble digesting beans. Be sure to soak the beans for at least fifteen hours before cooking them to facilitate digestion and help lessen the gassing caused when beans ferment in the intestines. This applies even to smaller beans such as lentils and split peas. Cook the beans slowly but thoroughly to soften the fiber without altering the protein.

In addition, you may want to eat bean sprouts instead, which are easier to digest and also contain more nutrients. Alfalfa sprouts, for example, are a nutrition powerhouse. They contain five times more Vitamin C than alfalfa seeds. Two ounces of sprouts a day will give you many vitamins and enzymes that might otherwise be missing from your diet. They also contain chlorophyll, which is considered to be a cleanser of the intestines and blood. Be sure to steam the bean sprouts briefly before eating them. The heat will neutralize any digestion inhibitors and other natural toxins contained in raw beans.

Common Carbohydrate Values

The calories and carbohydrate values for some common foods are listed in this chart. All figures are for edible portions of 3.5 ounces (100 grams). With some of these items, of course, you won't consume 100 grams at once. The higher the units, the more carbohydrates and/or sugar. A diabetic or hypoglycemic should try to stay away from ingesting any large units and preferably would eat no concentrated sugars—such as honey, corn syrup, dried figs, maple syrup, raisins, etc.

FOOD ITEM	CALORIES	UNITS
Sugar (beet or cane,) granulated	385	99.50
Brown sugar	373	96.40
Maple sugar	348	90.00
Puffed rice (cereal)	399	89.50
Cornflakes	386	85.30
Honey	304	82.30
Puffed wheat (cereal), with malt and sugar added	366	81.70
Carob flour	180	80.70
Buckwheat flour dark	333	79.50
Pastry flour (wheat)	364	79.40
Barley light	349	78.10
Rye flour, light	357	77.90
Raisins, uncooked	289	77.40
Whole wheat flour	364	76.90
Corn flour	368	76.80
Puffed oats (cereal)	397	75.20
Corn syrup (light or dark)	290	75.00
Cornmeal, whole	355	73.70
Rye, whole grain	334	73.40
Millet, whole grain	327	72.90

Dried apples, uncooked	275	71.80
Dried figs	274	69.10
Dried peaches, uncooked	262	68.30
Sorghum syrup	257	68.00
Dried prunes, uncooked	255	67.40
Dried pears	268	67.30
Dried apricots, uncooked	260	66.50
Light molasses	252	65.00
Maple syrup	252	65.00
Molasses, medium	232	60.00
Popcorn, cooked in oil	456	59.10
Rice bran	276	50.80
Wheat germ raw, commercially milled	363	46.70
Brewer's yeast, debittered	283	38.40
Whole milk, dry	502	38.20
Soybean flour, defatted	326	38.10
Sunflower seed flour, partially defatted	339	37.70
Torula yeast	277	37.00
Soybean flour, low fat	356	36.60
Grapefruit juice, frozen	145	34.60
Persimmons, native, raw	127	33.50
Sweet potatoes with skin, baked	141	32.50
Garlic cloves, raw	137	30.80
Almond meal, partially defatted	408	28.90
Soybean milk, powdered	429	28.00
Brown rice, cooked	119	25.50
Spaghetti, enriched, cooked until tender	111	23.00
Bananas, raw	85	22.20
Dried apricots, cooked, no sugar added	85	21.60
Red beans, dry, boiled and drained	118	21.40
Baked potatoes with skin	93	21.10
Corn on the cob	91	21.00
Split peas, cooked	115	20.80
Peanuts with skins, roasted	582	20.60
Pinenuts (pignolias)	635	20.50

Figs, raw	80	20.30
Sunflower seed kernels, dried	560	19.90
Almonds, dried	598	19.50
Cherries (sweet), raw	70	17.40
Grapes (European), raw	67	17.30
Potatoes with skin, boiled	76	17.10
Mangoes, raw	66	16.80
Filberts (hazelnuts)	634	16.70
Jerusalem artichokes, raw	7	16.70
Pomegranate pulp, raw	63	16.70
Spanish rice, homemade	87	16.60
Black raspberries, raw	73	15.70
Blueberries, raw	62	15.30
Pumpkin seeds, raw	553	15.00
Parsnips, cooked	66	14.90
Black walnuts	628	14.80
Acorn squash, baked	55	14.00
Pineapple, raw	52	13.70
Apricots raw	51	12.80
Orange, raw	49	12.20
Apple juice, canned or bottled	47	11.90
Hubbard squash, baked	50	11.70
Pinenuts, raw	552	11.60
Cranberries, raw	46	10.80
Grapefruit, raw	41	10.80
Butternut squash, boiled	41	10.40
Orange juice, frozen concentrate, unsweetened	45	10.30
Papayas, raw	39	10.00
Artichokes (globe or French), boiled and drained	44	9.90
Beets, raw	43	9.90
Carrots, raw	42	9.70
Peaches, raw	38	9.70
Greek olives	338	8.70
Onions, raw	38	8.70
Parsley, raw	44	8.50
Strawberries, raw	37	8.40
Brussels sprouts, raw	45	8.30

Scallions, raw	36	8.20
Honeydew melon	33	7.70
Okra, raw	36	7.60
Cantalope, raw	30	7.50
Collards, raw	45	7.50
Beets, cooked	32	7.20
Carrots, boiled and drained	31	7.10
Green beans, raw	32	7.10
Kohlrabi, raw	29	6.60
Onions, cooked	29	6.50
Brussels sprouts, cooked	36	6.40
Dandelion greens, cooked	33	6.40
Watermelon, raw	26	6.40
Broccoli, raw	32	5.90
Cider vinegar	14	5.90
Cabbage, raw	24	5.40
Green beans, boiled and drained	25	5.40
Soybean sprouts, raw	46	5.30
Turnips, boiled and drained	23	4.90
Green peppers (sweet), raw	22	4.80
Chard (Swiss), raw	25	4.60
Goat's milk	67	4.60
Broccoli, cooked	26	4.50
Mushrooms, raw	28	4.40
Spinach, raw	26	4.30
Radishes (Oriental, including daikon and Chinese), raw	19	4.20
Eggplant, boiled and drained	19	4.10
Asparagus spears, boiled and drained	20	3.60
Romaine lettuce	18	3.50
Zucchini, cooked	12	2.50
Tofu (soybean curd)	72	2.40
Tomatoes ripe, raw	22	.50
Cauliflower, raw	27	.20

Chapter 31

▼

Fat

Nearly a decade has passed since the American Heart Association recommended that we reduce our intake of saturated fats and cholesterol, but Americans still get nearly 45 percent of their total calories from fat. Although fat is a primary and necessary nutrient, a diet that includes too many high-fat foods will contribute to obesity and to cardiovascular and circulatory disorders. Oftentimes, a fatty plaque builds up in the arteries and causes atherosclerosis, which reduces the blood flow through the arteries and increases blood pressure.

Although it's important to monitor your fat intake, it's also important not to overreact and eliminate all foods that contain this nutrient from your diet. Some sources of fat are better than others, and there is no reason to abandon these nutritious foods. As with carbohydrates, the trick is to choose your fat sources wisely—and then eat them in the appropriate amounts.

The Need for Fat

The principal function of fat is to serve as a backup source of energy. It is deposited in adipose tissues throughout the body for this very purpose. Every gram of fat produces nine calories when it is oxidized, making it a potent and highly concentrated energy source. Carbohydrates and protein, by comparison, yield four calories per gram.

Small amounts of fat help the immune system to function properly by allowing us to use the fat-soluble Vitamins A, D, E, and K, which prevent viral infections. It is essential to the utilization of nutrients and the production of hormones, accounting for much of the body's chemistry in that capacity. Fat also keeps skin healthy and slows the aging process.

Finally, fat protects our heart, blood vessels, and internal organs from bruising, rupture, or hemorrhage. This padding not only serves as a shock absorber but also insulates the body to prevent heat loss. There should be enough fat to surround the organs without actually penetrating them. If too much intramuscular fat forms in the muscles and organs, you face a greater risk of heart disease, diabetes, and other disorders.

Saturated and Unsaturated Fats

Most of your fat intake should come from unsaturated fats, generally defined as ones that are liquid at room temperature. These fats come primarily from grains, legumes, seeds, nuts, and derivative oils, such as safflower, corn, sunflower, and soy oil.

Unsaturated fats provide the body with the essential fatty acids—linoleic acid, linolenic acid, and oleic acid—that control high blood pressure, monitor cell permeability, and give rise to prostaglandins. Even though these fatty acids are crucial for body functioning, consuming too many unsaturated fats can lead to liver damage, blood disorders, premature aging, and possibly even breast cancer. If your diet does not provide the nonessential fatty acids, the body will manufacture them itself.

Animal sources, such as meat and dairy products, provide the saturated fats that comprise half of the USDA's "basic four food groups." The carbon atom chains that compose these fats are saturated with hydrogen atoms; hence, the designation "saturated." These fats typically are solid at room temperature. They come from such foods as butter, lard, and the fatty part of chicken, fish, veal, lamb, pork, and beef (the visible marbled fat).

A word of caution: When shopping for unsaturated vegetable oil products, be wary of those that have been "hydrogenated." This process changes the oil from polyunsaturated to saturated and makes it into a solid product, such as salad oil, margarine, and egg and cream substitutes. The food label will tell you that the product was derived from polyunsaturates, but it may not tell you that it is now saturated.

Fat Requirements

People in the health field often disagree about what percentage of calories should come from fat, with recommendations ranging from as little as 10 percent to as much as 30 percent. Generally, fat should account for 15 percent of your calories, and 75 percent of these calories, in turn, should come from unsaturated fats. The remaining one-fourth can come from saturated fats. You should get all the fat your body needs from a balanced diet without having to take supplements.

Again, the unsaturated fats should come from the most natural sources possible—vegetables, grains, legumes, nuts, and seeds—and from cooking and salad oils. Avoid fats that have lost their nutritive value through food processing and chemical alteration. Fats in their natural state will provide the body with a necessary energy source and with Vitamin E, which serves as an antioxidant.

High-Fat Diets

The rationale behind a high-fat and high-protein diet (with a relatively low amount of carbohydrates) is that fat and protein will keep you feeling full for a long period of time while they are being digested. A fatty or high-protein meal takes four to six hours to digest in the stomach, thereby suppressing your appetite between meals. That's when many people overeat the wrong kinds of food—namely refined carbohydrates, such as soft drinks, doughnuts, and candy—and end up gaining weight.

By eliminating these snacks, the dieters can cut some four-hundred to nine-hundred calories per day and lose a pound of weight within a week. What these diets fail to recognize, however, is that regular exercise can do a lot more to control weight by heightening your metabolic functioning than cutting calories can accomplish on its own.

The Dangers of Fat

Deep-fried foods, such as french fries, fried fish, and doughnuts, can harm the body in a number of ways. First, they irritate the stomach and intestines because the foods are cooked in extremely hot, fatty oils that alter their chemical structure and create free fatty acids. Eventually, these foods can cause your intestines to become dysfunctional and lead to conditions such as colitis and spastic colon.

Deep-fried fats also slow down the digestive process. The enzymes in the stomach and intestines have a tougher time breaking down the fat once it is heated for a long period of time. Liquid fats, by comparison, go through the system much more easily. As a result, a fatty meal will sap you of energy. When the body must use a lot of energy to digest, absorb, and eliminate the foods you have eaten, your brain cannot draw the amount of blood and oxygen it needs. A person's ability to digest fats and protein also lessens with age as the secretion of hydrolyzing fat decreases. The gall bladder, which stores and secretes bile that helps to break down fats, may begin to function less well and inhibit fat digestion.

Remember that nearly all of the fat you consume is digested and utilized by the system. If you have too much fat in reserve and do not exercise on a regular basis, the muscles will begin to atrophy and fat will infiltrate the tissues. As fat takes the place of the sedentary muscles, you lose strength and stamina and open yourself up to more diseases and injuries.

Common Fat Values

The following chart lists the calories and unit value (in grams) for some common foods. All figures are for edible portions of 3.5 ounces (100 grams). With some of these foods, you won't consume 100 grams at once. Adjust your calculations accordingly.

FOOD ITEMS	CALORIES	UNITS
Lard	902	100.00
Butter	716	81.00

Margarine	720	81.00
Mayonnaise	718	79.90
Macadamia nuts	691	71.60
Pecans	687	71.20
Hickory nuts	673	68.70
Brazil nuts	654	66.90
Coconut meat dried, unsweetened	662	64.90
Walnuts	651	64.00
Filberts (hazelnuts)	634	62.40
Butternuts	629	61.20
Pinenuts	635	60.50
Italian salad dressing, commercial, regular	552	60.00
Black walnuts	628	59.30
Almonds dried	598	54.20
Pistachio nuts	594	53.70
Sesame seeds, dry, hulled	582	53.40
Peanuts with skins, roasted	582	48.70
Cashew nuts	561	45.70
Potato chips	568	39.80
Soybean flour	421	20.30
Eggs, fried	216	17.20

Chapter 32

▼

Proteins

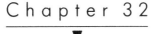

Simply put, protein is the substance of life. It provides the basic building materials for our cells, tissues, and organs and fuels nearly all of our metabolic functions. But this very importance has led many people—including athletes—to draw an incorrect conclusion regarding their protein intake. If protein is so important, they reason, then more must necessarily be better. Unfortunately, this leap in logic has resulted in an overconsumption of protein and an overdependence on meat in our diets.

The average American consumes about twice the amount of protein required by the body each day. The average intake is nearly 100 grams per day, while 45 to 50 grams would meet all of our needs. In addition, meat has long been the primary source of protein for most Americans even though other nutritious sources are readily available, including eggs, dairy products, legumes, grains, nuts, and seeds. People often overlook the value of these alternative sources because they have been conditioned to believe that meat must be the centerpiece of every meal.

A better approach is to recognize the very real need for protein in your diet but limit your intake to the correct amount for your body weight and to the most nutritious sources (consumed alone or combined with other foods to form a complete protein).

The Need for Protein

Protein is the foundation upon which our cells and, therefore, our bodies are built. It is second only to water in comprising our body weight. As such, protein plays a vital role in many body functions. We need it to grow properly; to maintain healthy bones, muscles, nerves, skin, and teeth; to metabolize our foods; and to sustain a proper blood count. The hemoglobin that supplies our cells with oxygen is made of protein.

The enzymes that fuel metabolism also are protein molecules. Without these enzymes, hundreds of metabolic reactions could not take place in the body. The liver could not synthesize carbohydrates, fats, proteins, and cholesterol, for example, and the cells could not store and release energy. Proteins combine with fat to form lipoproteins and transport fat through the bloodstream. They also serve as the building blocks of antibodies, which protect you from infection and disease.

Complete proteins, which contain all of the essential amino acids, must be eaten at every meal because the body cannot store protein. People who do not eat animal products must mix their foods to form a complete protein. When the amino acids are not present in the proper amounts, the cells cannot synthesize the proteins they need. Even one missing amino acid will prevent the protein from being constructed, just as one missing beam will prevent a building from going up. The amino acids also allow the body to utilize certain vitamins and minerals.

Protein Requirements

The amount of protein that you need will depend on your age, stage of growth, and physical condition. For the most part, adults require 0.9 grams of protein for each kilogram (2.2 pounds) of body weight. A 120-pound woman (54.5 kilograms), for example, requires 49 grams of protein per day, while a 170-pound man (77 kilograms) requires 69 grams.

The body needs more protein during the crucial growth stages of infancy, early childhood, and puberty. Other people who require more protein are pregnant and lactating women; people recovering from surgery and some types of infections, shock, and fever; hypoglycemics; and people experiencing stress. Likewise, vegetarians may need to increase their protein intake to compensate for the fact that plant sources have a slower absorption rate than meats. Conversely, people with such conditions as kidney disease may need less protein for a period of time.

The Essential Amino Acids

The twenty-three recognized amino acids are the basic substances from which the body makes proteins. While fifteen of these amino acids can be synthesized in the body, eight of them must be obtained from food. As a result, these eight are called "essential" amino acids. The other fifteen are called "nonessential" because the body can produce them.

Complete protein foods contain the correct amounts of all the essential amino acids, including threonine, valine, tryptophan, lysine, methionine, histidine, phenylalanine, and isoleucine. The body can become deficient in protein if we eat foods that lack one or more of the essential amino acids or if we simply fail to meet our protein requirements. The complete protein foods are eggs, meat, fish, fowl, and dairy products.

The body can only absorb and use protein if our food contains the correct proportions of each of the essential amino acids. The proportions found in eggs, for example, are considered to be ideal. Even foods that contain all eight amino acids are only partially complete if the proportions are incorrect. Therefore, foods that provide partially complete proteins must be eaten in combination with other foods that supplement the missing amino acids. These foods include brewer's yeast, wheat germ, tofu, peanuts, and certain micro-sea algae. The brewer's yeast can be sprinkled on cereal or blended with milk; wheat germ can be added to lentil burgers; tofu can be mixed with algae in salads; and peanut butter can be spread on whole-wheat bread.

Preparing Protein Foods

Generally, proteins are easiest to digest when they are cooked with moderate heat. Beans and legumes, for example, contain certain toxins that inhibit digestion unless they are cooked or sprouted. (Certain legumes contain even stronger toxins that must be neutralized by heat.) And some legumes have phytic acid in their husks that can bind zinc, calcium, and other minerals in the intestines, thereby causing deficiencies.

All grains contain this phytic acid as well, so they must be sprouted and baked with yeast or cooked thoroughly. To prevent a zinc or calcium deficiency, vegetarians will need to take supplements or eat more foods that contain these minerals, such as egg yolks, peas, seafood, corn, carrots, and yeast. Meat, for its part, must be cooked slowly but completely to neutralize any microorganisms it contains. Pork, in particular, must be cooked thoroughly to prevent trichinosis, which may be caused by a parasite it contains.

In general, however, animal and plant proteins should not be overheated. Doing so can create "cross-linkages," just as a permanent wave curls hair. These cross-linkages complicate the process by which enzymes break down proteins into simple, digestible amino acids. Hence, fried or overcooked protein foods should be avoided. And milk and related products should never be heated past the boiling point. People who have trouble digesting milk can try cultured products such as yogurt and buttermilk. The healthy microorganisms in these products will predigest the lactose sugar that bothers many people and change it to an easily digested lactic acid.

The Dangers of Too Much or Too Little

It's important to get the right amount of protein in your diet, without tipping the scale too far in either direction. People who eat too many partially complete proteins, for example, will be deficient in certain amino acids needed for growth. They should supplement these foods with others that complement the amino acid content.

Consider the millions of poor people whose diet consists primarily of bread or cereal for prolonged periods of time. The wheat, on its own, simply does not promote adequate growth during the children's formative years. Likewise, adults who get their protein from a few limited sources are likely to hinder their immune system because proteins form the antibodies that fight infections. One only needs to look at the condition of their skin and hair to see that a deficiency exists.

In short, incomplete proteins cannot support life. They do an inadequate job of building new cells and tissues or replacing those that have become old. The diseases that result from a protein deficiency, such as marasmus and kwashiorkor, often crop up among people who attempt to live on incomplete proteins. This is true of South Americans, who primarily eat beans and corn; Africans, who eat millet; and Asians, who eat rice and some legumes.

At the other end of the spectrum are people who consume too much protein, often because they mistakenly believe that protein foods are low in calories. To the contrary, the beef, pork, and other protein sources recommended by high-protein, low-carbohydrate diets are loaded with calories. These meats contain fat, after all, so they will yield four calories for every gram of protein and 9 calories for every gram of fat. As much as 50 percent of filet mignon is fat, for example, which means that one portion alone can have 400 to 500 calories.

As stated earlier, these misleading diets operate on the theory that a high-protein meal, which takes a long time to digest, will prevent you from getting hungry between meals and snacking on highly refined and sugary carbohydrates. So the large amount of calories you consume during the meal simply stops you from eating other high-calorie foods for several hours.

What does your body do with the excess protein? At first it simply burns it for energy, a taxing but relatively harmless metabolic process. Eventually, however, excess protein can begin to overstress the kidneys by releasing too much ammonium into the body through the process of deaminization. The ammonium turns to urea and must be excreted through the kidneys along with excess sodium because meats contain more salt than vegetables. Overconsumption of protein can also cause edema and dehydration; people who eat a lot of protein typically require extra water.

Other potential problems include arteriosclerosis and heart disease, because animal foods have more saturated fats and cholesterol than vegetables. People who eat both meat proteins and refined carbohydrates put themselves at an even greater risk for these conditions. In most cases, it's better to eat more complex carbohydrates, vegetable proteins, and fruits than to begin a high-protein diet. By modifying your behavior and exercising regularly, you can not only lose weight but also enhance health life in other ways.

Common Protein Values

The protein values for some common vegetarian foods are listed in this chart. The figures are based on an edible portion of 3.5 ounces (100 grams). In some cases, you will not eat 100 grams in one serving. Adjust your calculations accordingly.

FOOD ITEM	CALORIES	UNITS
Soybean protein	322	74.90
Soybean flour, defatted	326	47.00
Sunflower seed flour, partially defatted	339	45.20
Soybean milk, powder	429	41.80
Wheat flour 45% gluten, 55% patent	378	41.40
Soybean flour, high fat	380	41.20
Rice cereal, with casein	382	40.00
Almond meal, partially defatted	408	39.50
Brewer's yeast, debittered	283	38.80
Torula yeast	277	38.60
Skim milk, dry, regular	363	35.90
Pinenuts (pignolias)	552	31.10
Wheat germ, toasted	391	30.00
Pumpkin and squash seed kernals, dried	553	29.00
Peanut butter	581	27.80
Swiss cheese (domestic), unprocessed	370	27.50
Wheat germ, raw, comercially milled	363	26.60
Peanuts with skins, roasted	582	26.20
Cheddar cheese, unprocessed	398	25.00
Brick cheese	370	22.20
Blue cheese or Roquefort cheese	369	21.50
Black walnuts	628	20.50
Pistachio nuts	594	19.30
Shredded oats (cereal)	279	18.80
Sesame seeds, dry, hulled	582	18.20
Cashew nuts	561	17.20
Cottage cheese, uncreamed	86	17.00
Oatmeal (baby food), commercial	375	16.50
Rye flour, dark	327	16.30
Flaked oats (cereal)	397	14.90
Walnuts	651	14.80
Brazil nuts	654	14.30

Eggs, fried	216	13.80
Cottage cheese, creamed	106	13.60
Rice bran	276	13.30
Whole wheat flour	333	13.30
Rye wafers whole grain	344	13.00
Eggs, hard-boiled	163	12.90
Popcorn, plain	386	12.70
Filberts (hazelnuts)	634	12.60
Rye, whole grain	334	12.10
Puffed oats (cereal)	397	11.90
Buckwheat flour, whole grain	335	11.70
Whole wheat bread, toasted	287	10.80
Miso (fermented soybean product)	171	10.50
Whole wheat bread, commercial	243	10.50
Bulgur	357	10.40
Bran flakes cereal	303	10.20
Wheat flakes (cereal)	354	10.20
Barley, pearled	348	9.60
Cornmeal, whole ground, unbolted	355	9.20
Pecans	687	9.20
Soybeans, canned, drained solids	103	9.00
Cowpeas, boiled	130	8.90
Cornmeal, whole ground, self-rising	347	8.50
Lima beans, dry, boiled and drained	138	8.20
Potato flour	351	8.00
Split peas, cooked	115	8.00
Tofu (soybean curd)	72	7.80
Baby lima beans frozen, boiled and drained	118	7.40
Corn, rice, and wheat flakes (cereal)	389	7.40
White rice, parboiled	369	7.40
Coconut meat, dried, unsweetened	662	7.20
Soybean sprouts, raw	46	6.20
Mung bean sprouts, raw	35	3.80
Buttermilk, cultured	36	3.60
Collard greens, boiled	33	3.60
Parsley, raw	44	3.60
Skim milk	36	3.60
Whole milk	65	3.50

Soybean milk, fluid	33	3.40
Yogurt, made from partially skimmed milk	50	3.40
Goat's milk	67	3.20

Chapter 33

▼

Vitamins

Vitamins are organic compounds that activate and regulate the body's metabolic functioning through the formation of enzymes. While they have no caloric value, vitamins are essential for life. They aid in the processes of converting food to energy, forming bone and tissue, and building major body structures.

All vitamins fall into two general categories: water soluble and oil soluble. The water-soluble vitamins, including B-Complex, C, and the bioflavonoids, must be replenished daily because the body cannot store them. The oil-soluble vitamins, including A, D, E, and K, are absorbed and stored in the body with the help of oil.

What follows is a description of each vitamin's uses in the body, its various food sources, the signs of deficiency, and the Recommended Daily Allowances (RDAs), which generally are set by the Food and Nutrition Board of the National Academy of Science or the National Research Council. Quantities are given as grams, some portion thereof, or international units (I.U.s).

Vitamin A

▶ Uses: Vitamin A is needed for the growth and repair of body tissues. It helps to maintain the skin and protect the mucous membranes of the lungs, throat, mouth, and nose. Vitamin A is essential for maintenance of the immune system. It also plays a role in protein digestion and protects the linings of the kidneys, bladder, and digestive tract. Finally, it helps to form rich blood, maintain good eyesight, and build strong bones and teeth.

► Sources: Green leafy vegetables such as spinach, beet greens, and broccoli, carrots, eggs, whole milk, and milk products. Although animal livers also have concentrated amounts of Vitamin A, this waste-filtering organ also will contain any hormones or chemicals to which the animal was exposed.

► Signs of deficiency: One of the first warning signs is night blindness, characterized by the eyes' inability to adjust to darkness. Other signs include fatigue, loss of appetite and the sense of smell, unhealthy skin, and diarrhea.

► RDA: 5,000 I.U. daily for adults. People who suffer from disease or trauma and pregnant and lactating women may need more.

B-Complex Vitamins

These eleven water-soluble vitamins work as a team to release the nutrients in carbohydrates, fats, and proteins and convert them to energy. The team works harmoniously in every cell of the body when each of the vitamins is present in the proper proportion. Foods, such as nutritional yeast, eggs, liver, seed germs, meat, and vegetables, contain a lot of the B-Complex vitamins. An increase in muscular work (i.e., running or participating in other endurance sports) will require an increase in these vitamins.

Vitamin B_1 (Thiamine)

► Uses: This vitamin is essential to nerve functioning and normal metabolism. It converts carbohydrates to glucose, the sole source of energy for the nervous system and the brain. It also keeps the heart firm and resilient.

▶ Sources: Such foods as whole grains, legumes, fish, and poultry.

▶ Signs of deficiency: Since a Vitamin B$_1$ deficiency can weaken the insulating sheath that protects certain nerve fibers, the nerves may become hypersensitive, causing irritability, sluggishness, forgetfulness, and apathy. If the degeneration continues, the nerves in the legs may become weak and cause pain in the legs and feet. The end result could be paralysis. A deficiency also may lead to constipation, indigestion, anorexia, and heart trouble due to increased blood circulation.

▶ RDA: 1.0 milligram for adult females; 1.4 milligrams for men. Your intake should be increased if you perspire heavily, drink tea or coffee, take antibiotics, or have a fever or are experiencing a lot of stress. Some nutritionists recommend that athletes take 10 to 20 milligrams daily.

Vitamin B$_2$ (Riboflavin)

▶ Uses: Vitamin B$_2$ promotes proper growth and tissue repair and enhances cell respiration. It helps to release energy from food and contributes to good digestion, steady nerves, normal vision, and the assimilation of iron. It is essential to the proper operation of the entire glandular system, especially the adrenal glands that help to control stress.

▶ Sources: Dairy products, meat, fish, poultry, nutritional yeast, whole grains, leafy green vegetables, and soybean.

▶ Signs of deficiency: The tongue turns a purplish red and becomes inflamed or shiny. Other symptoms include cracks at the corners of the lips, hypersensitivity to light, bloodshot eyes, blurred vision, greasy skin, itchiness, depression, insomnia, and reduced mental alertness.

▶ RDA: 1.6 milligrams daily for adult males; 1.2 milligrams for females.

► Uses: This vitamin is vital for every body cell. It comprises the basic material for two enzyme systems and helps convert sugar and fat into energy.

► Sources: Organ meats, salmon, tuna, leafy green vegetables, wheat germ, brewer's yeast, beans, peas and dried figs, prunes, and dates.

► Signs of deficiency: Many of the crucial metabolic functions may cease to take place. Low levels of Vitamin B_3 may lead to mental illness and pellagra, which causes disorders of the skin and intestinal tract.

► RDA: 13 milligrams daily for adult females; 18 milligrams for men. An excess of Vitamin B_3 may cause the muscles to use glycogen more quickly and thereby result in fatigue.

Vitamin B₅

► Uses: Vitamin B_5 converts carbohydrates, fats, and proteins to energy and work in every body cell. It serves as an anti-stress agent and manufactures antibodies that fight infections in the blood.

► Sources: Many common foods such as eggs, whole grains, beans, peanuts, and organ meats.

► Signs of deficiency: The warning signs include a strong tendency to infections and illness, vomiting and abdominal pain, leg cramps and other nerve disorders, depression and insomnia.

► RDA: Not yet established; the Food and Nutrition Board suggests 5 to 10 milligrams daily for adults.

Vitamin B₆ (Pyridoxine)

► Uses: Vitamin B_6 nourishes the central nervous system, aids in the production of red blood cells and hemoglobin, and controls sodium and potassium levels in the blood. It helps to manufacture DNA and RNA, the nucleic acids that contain your genetic code for cell growth, repair, and multiplication. It also prevents infections. Vitamin B_6 is vital for endurance sports because it assists in the initial breakdown of glycogen

► Sources: Brewer's yeast, brown rice, bananas, pears, beef, pork liver, and seafood such as salmon and herring.

► Signs of deficiency: As with a Vitamin B_2 deficiency, the signs include nervousness, irritability, weakness, insomnia, dermatitis, and similar changes in skin condition.

► RDA: 2 milligrams per every 100 grams of protein consumed.

Vitamin B_{12} (Cyanocobalamin)

► Uses: Vitamin B_{12}, the most complex of the B vitamins, contributes to the functioning of every cell. It is especially important to cells in the bone marrow, intestinal tract, and nervous system. Vitamin B_{12} also helps to monitor body weight and prevent fats from depositing in the liver.

► Sources: Fermented soybean products such a tempeh, nonfat dry milk, poultry, and meat. Because the natural form of B_{12} is manufactured by microorganisms, vegetables and fruits typically do not contain it.

► Signs of deficiency: Symptoms include motor and mental abnormalities, rapid heartbeat or cardiac pain, facial swelling, jaundice, weakness and fatigue, hair or weight loss, depression, and an impaired memory.

► RDA: 30 milligrams daily.

Folic Acid

► Uses: This vitamin contributes to brain and nervous system functioning. It is a crucial component of spinal and extracellular fluid. Folic acid also helps to convert amino acids and is used in the manufacturing of DNA and RNA.

► Sources: Brewer's yeast, dark green leafy vegetables, wheat germ, oysters, salmon, and chicken.

► RDA: 400 milligrams is recommended because the body needs relatively minuscule amounts of folic acid. The elderly, pregnant women, and people who suffer from any nervous disorder may need more.

Para-Aminobenzoic Acid (PABA)

► Uses: PABA, a component of folic acid, acts as a coenzyme in the metabolism of protein. It helps to manufacture healthy blood cells and can aid in the healing of skin disorders. PABA also protects your skin against sunburn by absorbing the portions of the ultraviolet spectrum that are known to cause burns and even skin cancer.

► Sources: Eggs, brewer's yeast, molasses, wheat germ, and whole grains.

► Signs of deficiency: The signals include digestive trouble, nervous tension, emotional instability, and blotchy skin.

► RDA: Not yet established.

Choline

► Uses: Choline serves as a fat remover in all cellular membranes and helps to regulate cholesterol levels. It plays an important role in liver functioning and aids in the construction and maintenance of a healthy nervous system.

► Sources: Wheat germ and bran, beans, egg yolks, brewer's yeast, whole grains, nuts, lecithin, meat, and fish.

► Signs of deficiency: The liver will be unable to process any type of fat. The fatty deposits in the liver will hinder its normal filtering process. Muscle weakness and excessive scarring also may be present.

► RDA: The body produces it own supply with protein and other B vitamins. While a daily requirement has not been set, the average daily intake is estimated at 500 to 900 milligrams.

Inositol

▶ Uses: Inositol emulsifies fat, thereby preventing cholesterol buildup and normalizing fat metabolism. It also serves as a natural tranquilizer of sorts by reducing anxiety.

▶ Sources: Wheat germ, brewer's yeast, whole grains, nuts, oranges, and molasses. The body makes inositol with the help of bacterial or intestinal flora found in the intestinal tract. Therefore, the best way to get a sufficient amount is to maintain a healthy intestinal tract.

▶ Signs of deficiency: Symptoms include insomnia, hair loss, a high cholesterol level, and cirrhosis of the liver.

▶ RDA: Not yet established.

Biotin

▶ Uses: Biotin promotes the growth of healthy hair, skin, bone marrow, and glands. It also assists in the production of energy from fatty acids, carbohydrates, and amino acids. It is vital to the production of glycogen.

▶ Sources: The body manufactures biotin in the intestinal tract. Other sources include such foods as eggs, cheese, and nuts.

▶ Signs of deficiency: While a biotin deficiency is rare, the signs include fatigue, depression, skin disorders, slow healing of wounds, muscular pain, anorexia, sensitivity to cold temperatures, and a high blood cholesterol level.

▶ RDA: 150 to 300 micrograms daily.

Vitamin C

▶ Uses: Vitamin C contributes to a wide variety of body functions. It strengthens the immune system, reduces cholesterol levels, fights stress, promotes fertility, maintains mental health, and prolongs the life span. Vitamin C combats toxic substances in our food, air, and water. It also protects the body against cardiovascular disease and various forms of cancer. Vitamin C is needed to build collagen, the substance that holds together the body's connective tissue; athletes have an increased need for collagen synthesis and tissue repair.

▶ Sources: Important sources include whole oranges and other citrus fruits, sprouts, berries, tomatoes, sweet potatoes, and leafy green vegetables.

▶ Signs of deficiency: Warning signs include bleeding gums, a tendency to bruise easily, shortness of breath, impaired digestion, nosebleeds, swollen or painful joints, anemia, a lowered resistance to infections, and slow healing of wounds and fractures.

▶ RDA: The official daily dosage is 45 milligrams. Some nutritionists, however, believe that doses of up to 10 grams daily will help to prevent serious illnesses and reduce the risk of cancer. People with a greater need for Vitamin C include the elderly, dieters, smokers, heavy drinkers, pregnant and lactating women, people experiencing stress, and those who use medications, including oral contraceptives.

Vitamin D

▶ Uses: This oil-soluble vitamin helps the body to utilize calcium and phosphorus in forming strong bones and teeth and healthy skin. It is essential to the functioning of the kidneys and nervous system as well.

▶ Sources: Sunshine is a primary source; others include fortified milk and butter, egg yolks, fish liver oils, and seafood such as sardines, salmon, tuna, and herring.

▶ Signs of deficiency: Common symptoms include brittle and fragile bones, soft bones and teeth, pale skin, some forms of arthritis, insomnia, irregular heartbeat, and an abnormally slow healing of injuries.

▶ RDA: At least 400 I.U. daily. More may be needed to build the body's resistance to bone disease, but megadoses of this storable vitamin are not recommended.

Vitamin E

▶ Uses: Vitamin E serves primarily as an antioxidant. It protects fatty acids from destruction, maintains the integrity of all body cells and promotes the health of muscles, cells, blood, and skin. It also defends against respiratory infections and disease. Vitamin E has a bacterial response that makes it an excellent tonic for burns. Its antioxidant effects are believed to supply large amounts of fats for metabolism, which provides the body with extra energy for muscle contractions.

▶ Sources: Wheat germ and wheat germ oil, leafy plant foods eaten with cold pressed oils, whole grains, seeds, nuts, and fertile eggs.

▶ Signs of deficiency: Warning signs include facial swelling, ankle and leg swelling, poor skin condition, muscle cramps, abnormal heartbeat, and respiratory difficulties.

▶ RDA: Nutritionists and doctors recommend 30 to 400 I.U. daily for adults, unless an existing condition requires larger amounts.

Vitamin K

▶ Uses: This oil-soluble vitamin helps the blood to clot properly and promotes proper bone development and functioning.

▶ Sources: Microflora in the large intestines produce Vitamin K. Yogurt and other fermented dairy and soy products can assist in this process. Other sources include green leafy plants such as spinach, kale, cauliflower, broccoli, and cabbage.

► Signs of deficiency: One primary symptom is a tendency to bruise easily, but this can be a sign of other nutritional deficiencies as well.

► RDA: The precise daily minimum needed is not known, and over-the-counter supplements are not available.

Bioflavonoids

► Uses: This group of water-soluble substances ensures that capillaries are strong and properly functioning. In conjunction with Vitamin C, they help to produce collagen in the capillary walls. The bioflavonoids also protect cells against viruses and bacteria.

► Sources: Ordinarily, bioflavonoids are found in foods that contain Vitamin C, including grapes, rosehips, prunes, oranges, lemon juice, cherries, black currants, plums, parsley, cabbage, apricots, peppers, papaya, cantaloupe, tomatoes, and broccoli.

► Signs of deficiency: The signs include bleeding gums and easily bruised skin.

► RDA: Not yet established. Most nutritionists agree that adults can take 500 milligrams daily.

▼

Chapter 34

Minerals

Although minerals constitute just 5 percent of body weight, they serve as essential building material for the blood, nerve cells, muscle, tissue, bones, and teeth. They also prompt many of the body's biological reactions and help to maintain the delicate balance of body fluids. The minerals perform various types of work that are interrelated in the body, so that the actions of any one will affect the functioning of others.

As with the section on vitamins, this chapter centers on the uses, sources, signs of deficiency, and recommended daily intake for each of eleven minerals. For the most part, the body needs only small amounts of these substances.

Calcium

► Uses: As the body's chief mineral, calcium is the primary component of bones, teeth, and the fluid that bathes body cells. It is used in the production of hormones, the release of adrenaline and noradrenaline into the bloodstream to combat stress, and the stimulation of enzymes. Without it, the body cannot store glucose as glycogen in the muscles. Along with several other minerals, calcium helps to maintain the pH level of blood and protect it against overacidity.

► Sources: Milk, dairy products such as yogurt, buttermilk, acidophilus milk, and kefir (which are more easily absorbed by the body), and cheeses. Sesame seeds, torula yeast, carob flour, and sea vegetables contain smaller amounts.

► Signs of deficiency: The warning signs include nervousness, depression, headaches, and insomnia. Without a steady supply of calcium, your bones and teeth would not remain hard, the brain would not function properly, the muscles could not store energy, and the digestive, immune, and circulatory systems would suffer. An inadequate supply of calcium may also lead to the creation of calcium deposits as the body removes the substance from its reserves and lodges it in soft tissue.

► RDA: 800 milligrams daily for healthy adults; 1,200 milligrams for pregnant and lactating women.

Chromium

► Uses: This mineral is vital to the functioning of the brain, liver, and heart. It also contributes to glucose metabolism and the production of protein. The white blood cells need chromium to help fight bacteria, viruses, toxins, arthritis, cancer, and premature aging. The adrenal glands must have sufficient chromium to counteract stress.

► Sources: Whole-wheat flour, brewer's yeast, nuts, black pepper, whole-grain cereals (excluding rye and corn), fresh fruit juices, dairy products, root vegetables, legumes, leafy vegetables, and mushrooms.

► Signs of deficiency: These include fatigue, dizziness, anxiety, insomnia, a craving for alcohol, blurred vision, depression, and panic. Without chromium, insulin cannot transport glucose from the bloodstream to the cells, and the liver cannot properly remove excess fat from the blood. Rapid premature aging may result from a deficiency as well, because protein production will be seriously impaired.

► RDA: None has been set officially, but trace mineral experts suggest a daily dosage of 200 micrograms.

Iodine

► Uses: Iodine is crucial to the production of thyroxin, the hormone that controls the speed at which your blood takes food from the intestines to the cells to be used as energy. It is also important to the functioning of the heart, immune system, and protein synthesis.

► Sources: Fresh seafood, garlic, sea vegetables such as hiziki, wakame, kelp, and dulse, dried mushrooms, leafy greens, celery, tomatoes, radishes, carrots, and onions.

► Signs of deficiency: Symptoms include poor complexion, unhealthy hair, teeth, and nails, and a sluggish feeling. The energy mechanism and metabolic process of the cells would be seriously impaired without an adequate supply of iodine. A child could not grow properly and healthy adult tissue could not be maintained. Your resistance to infection and the metabolism of fat in the bloodstream would be impaired if an iodine deficiency existed.

► RDA: 150 micrograms; some nutritionists believe that an intake of 300 micrograms is needed to prevent serious thyroid disorders.

Iron

► Uses: Because iron carries oxygen, you cannot live without it. It is needed for proper functioning of the hemoglobin in the red blood cells, the myoglobin in the muscles, and the enzymes linked to energy release.

► Sources: Animal livers (although any chemicals or hormones concentrated in the organs will be consumed as well), egg yolks (which contain more iron than muscle meats), leafy green vegetables, dried beans, peaches, apricots, dates, prunes, cherries, figs, raisins, and blackstrap molasses.

► Signs of deficiency: Warning signs include chronic fatigue, shortness of breath, headaches, pale skin, and opaque or brittle nails. An iron deficiency may lead to certain types of anemia that can hinder a runner's athletic performance and cause other health problems.

► RDA: 10 milligrams for adult men and 18 milligrams for women; pregnant women require 30 milligrams or more.

Magnesium

► Uses: This mineral plays a critical role in the cellular metabolic process, the manufacture of protein, and the production of hormones. It is one of the body's most important coenzymes. Magnesium contributes to the muscular, cellular, nervous, digestive, reproductive, blood, and immune systems.

► Sources: Leafy green vegetables, nuts, seeds, avocados, turnips, whole grains, legumes, organic eggs, raw milk, fruits and natural sweets such as carob, honey, and blackstrap molasses.

► Signs of deficiency: An irregular heartbeat is a primary sign. Hair loss and easily broken nails also signal a deficiency. Some consequences of a magnesium deficiency include the impairment of the immune response, muscle functioning, digestion, and protein production. Without magnesium, your bones would be too soft to support you, and you could not store energy, synthesize sex hormones, or prevent blood from clotting.

► RDA: 350 milligrams is the official quantity, but 450 to 650 milligrams may actually be needed to optimize health.

Manganese

► Uses: This trace mineral takes an active role in protein production and in promoting the correct structure of bones, teeth, cartilage, and tendons. It helps to form new blood cells in the bone marrow and transmit nerve impulses in the brain. Manganese also assists in the metabolism of blood sugar and fats and in the production of sex hormones.

► Sources: Nuts, seeds, whole grains, leafy green vegetables (when grown organically in mineral-rich soil), rhubarb, broccoli, carrots, potatoes, peas, beans, pineapple, blueberries, raisins, cloves, and ginger.

► Signs of deficiency: Blood sugar disorders and sexual dysfunction may be linked to a manganese deficiency. Other possible complications include myasthenia gravis, a slow deterioration of muscle health, and an inhibited protein production and carbohydrate/fat metabolism.

► RDA: Not yet established; trace mineral experts recommend up to 7 milligrams daily.

Phosphorus

► Uses: Phosphorus works in the bones, teeth, nerves, muscles, brain, liver, eyes, and the metabolic, cellular, digestive, and circulatory systems. It is an essential ingredient of your DNA and RNA. It also helps to balance the pH of body fluids and to supply energy to the muscles through carbohydrate oxidation, which makes it particularly important for runners.

► Sources: Most foods contain phosphorus, and those who eat a lot of refined foods may get too much of this mineral. Sources include meat, poultry, fish, eggs, dairy products, whole grains, nuts and seeds, legumes, celery, cabbage, carrots, cauliflower, string beans, cucumber, chard, pumpkin, and fruits.

► Signs of deficiency: Phosphorus deficiencies are rare. When a deficiency does occur, it could cause an anemia that results from abnormalities in the cellular membranes and an impaired resistance to bacteria and viruses.

► RDA: 800 milligrams for adults; 1,200 milligrams for pregnant and lactating women.

Potassium

▶ Uses: Potassium works with sodium to form an electrical pump that speeds nutrients to all body cells and carries out waste. It is vital to the functioning of the digestive and endocrine systems, muscles, brain, and nerves. It also helps to maintain the correct acid/alkaline balance of body fluids.

▶ Sources: Leafy green vegetables, bananas, cantaloupe, avocados, dates, prunes, dried apricots, raisins, whole grains, beans, legumes, nuts and seeds. In general, plant foods are far richer sources of this mineral than animal foods.

▶ Signs of deficiency: Common symptoms include a long healing time for injuries and a "worn out" quality to skin and other tissues. Other signs are lethargy, insomnia, severe constipation, intestinal spasms, tissue swelling, thinning hair, and malfunctioning muscles.

▶ RDA: Ordinarily, a proper diet will supply the necessary potassium. Runners, however, may require extra amounts because they lose the mineral through sweating. The consumption of two to four grams daily will replace the amount lost in urine, and runners can eat more potassium-rich foods during periods of intense training.

Selenium

▶ Uses: This mineral serves primarily as an antioxidant by protecting the cells from destruction of oxygen. It contributes to the enzyme system, protein production, and the manufacture of prostaglandins, which control blood pressure and clotting. Selenium also protects the eyes from cataracts and the artery walls from plaque.

▶ Sources: Animal foods, eggs (which also contain the sulphur that promotes selenium absorption and utilization), and vegetable sources such as whole grains, mushrooms, asparagus, broccoli, onions, and tomatoes. Animal foods generally provide more selenium than plant foods.

► Signs of deficiency: The signals include a lack of energy, accelerated angina, and the development of degenerative disease. A deficiency can also cause blood sugar disorders, liver necrosis, arthritis, anemia, heavy metal poisoning, muscular dystrophy, and cancer.

► RDA: An official level has not been set, but the Food and Nutrition Board suggests 150 micrograms daily.

Sodium

► Uses: Sodium works with potassium to deliver nutrients to the cells and remove waste products. It regulates cellular fluid pressure, which, in turn, affects blood pressure. Sodium is vital to the nerves' ability to transmit impulses to muscles and the muscles' ability to contract. It works with other nutrients to control the varying degrees of pH balance throughout the body. Sodium also helps to produce hydrochloric acid for digestion, pump glucose into the bloodstream, and keep calcium suspended in the bloodstream so that it is available to meet the tissues' needs.

► Sources: Nearly all types of food, including water, contain this mineral. Refined foods contain enormous amounts of sodium.

► Signs of deficiency: Sodium deficiency is uncommon. When it does occur, it is typically caused by stressful situations, such as exposure to toxic chemicals, infections, digestive problems, allergies, and injuries. Symptoms include wrinkles, sunken eyes, flatulence, diarrhea, nausea, vomiting, confusion, fatigue, low blood pressure, irritability, difficult breathing, and heightened allergies.

► RDA: The body needs 200 to 600 milligrams to function, but most people consume 7,000 to 22,000 milligrams daily. Excessive amounts of sodium can lead to serious problems, such as hypertension, stress, liver damage, muscular weakness, and pancreas disease.

▶ Uses: This mineral participates in the production of growth and sex hormones and the utilization of insulin. As a coenzyme, it initiates many important activities and sparks energy sources. Zinc contributes to homeostatic functions by maintaining the blood's proper acidity, producing necessary histamine, removing excess toxic metals, and aiding the kidneys in maintaining a healthy balance of minerals. Zinc also works in the protein production system, circulatory system, blood cells, liver, kidneys, muscles, bones, joints, immune system, nerves, and eyes.

▶ Sources: Eggs, poultry, seafood, organ meats, peas, soybeans, mushrooms, whole grains, and most nuts and seeds, particularly pumpkin seeds.

▶ Signs of deficiency: The signals include an impaired sense of taste or smell, acne, and psoriasis. Stretch marks are an indication that the elastin fibers that make your skin smooth and springy are not getting enough zinc. Other signs are an abnormal wearing away of tooth enamel, opaque fingernails, brittle hair, and bleeding gums.

▶ RDA: 20 to 25 milligrams.

Chapter 35

▼

The Body's Use of Fuel

The body draws its supply of energy from three sources: (1) carbohydrates, which are stored as glycogen in the muscles and liver; (2) fats, which float in the blood as free fatty acids and are stored in fat cells as tryglycerides; and (3) protein, which the liver converts to fat that is stored in the tissues.

All three forms of stored, or potential, energy can be used as a fuel after they have been oxidized and broken down into their component sugars and fatty acids. Each source requires a different amount of oxygen to supply the kinetic energy needed for movement. Carbohydrates need small amounts of oxygen to burn, while fat requires large amounts.

When you first begin to run or exercise, the body receives a limited amount of oxygen. As a result, it uses glycogen as 90 percent of its free fuel source. After ten minutes have passed, however, you will be getting more oxygen by taking more frequent and deeper breaths. The body begins to burn fat in the form of free fatty acids; some of these are floating in the blood and others are mobilized and converted from the tryglycerides stored in fat cells. The blood transports the free fatty acids to the muscles to be used as fuel.

These fats supply about 70 percent of the body's energy. The other 30 percent comes from the glycogen in muscles and the liver, which stores the fuel for about twelve hours. If you replenish your supply by eating carbohydrates, you will have enough energy to complete four hours of aerobic exercise. After that, the 30 percent glycogen component has been drained from the muscles and liver.

If the body's demand for energy continues after its glycogen and free fatty acids have been depleted, protein will be used as fuel. To do so, however, the body must break down its own tissue and convert it to energy. Therefore, protein is an extremely inefficient form of fuel. The body typically uses it as a last resort, such as when a person is fasting.

Chapter 36

▼

Supplements for Marathon Runners

There's no denying that a person will undergo enormous physical and psychological stress when training for and participating in a long-distance race. In essence, training for a marathon is not a *healthy* endeavor. It places wear and tear on the muscles and joints, depletes the protein storage in muscles, and taxes the immune system. Therefore, marathon training requires enormous amounts of energy and superior functioning of the body's muscle-mass retention, fat-burning capabilities, insulin regulation, and immune mechanism.

Considering the tremendous demands being placed on the body, it follows that the marathon runner should consider the use of various nutrient supplements in his or her diet. Supplementation is not a popular concept among the medical establishment, which maintains that the Recommended Daily Allowances (RDAs) provide sufficient nutrients for athletic endeavors. But we believe that the conventional wisdom simply does not account for the super-stressing effects that intensive training has on the body systems. We would question whether the top marathon runners have performed at their level with the standard supply of nutrients available from the average diet.

In previous chapters, we discussed the basic nutritional requirements for any person who exercises regularly to enhance his or her health. The importance of a well-rounded diet that includes appropriate amounts of all the major nutrients cannot be overstated. But in this chapter, we look specifically at some of the nutrients and food factors that may be required in excess of the RDA by athletes who are training for long-distance events. These include vitamins, minerals, and a variety of amino acids that contribute to aerobic performance.

Simply put, the use of supplements allows you to optimize your performance by optimizing your nutrition. It's like taking a four-cylinder car, which is functional but not especially powerful, and souping it up so that it can surpass the performance goals it was originally designed to meet. In the same way, the body can only do so much with the level of nutrients provided by the food we eat. By taking the appropriate supplements, we can soup up the many internal systems that drive our performance during a long-distance, endurance event.

Traditional sports medicine has taken a conservative view of this approach to supplementation. Many books on the role of nutrition in athletic performance will warn you off the use of any supplements unless they are needed to compensate for a specific deficiency. An athlete who is found to be low in iron, for example, would take an iron supplement to correct the problem. Indeed, the usual approach to supplementation is to identify a person's deficiencies and then raise his or her intake of those nutrients to the RDA.

In the National Association for Sports and Physical Education's *Nutrition for Sports Success*, for example, the authors express the prevailing wisdom about supplementation with the following statement: "A varied diet, sufficient in the amount to satisfy the energy needs of an active athlete, will provide adequate vitamins and minerals. Many of today's foods are 'fortified' with vitamins and minerals, thus adding to daily intake. If vitamin and mineral supplements are used, a single daily multivitamin (with or without minerals) that provides a maintenance level (100% of the RDA for each nutrient) is preferable to therapeutic level supplements (provide greater than 100% of the RDA)."

Likewise, this school of thought maintains that athletes can get all the amino acids they need by meeting the RDA for protein. In *Nutrition and Exercise*, for instance, Vernon R. Young draws this conclusion from studies that examined the relationship between exercise and protein/amino acid requirements: "Therefore, from this set of observations, it is reasonable to conclude that at intakes of protein amounting to about 1–1.5g/kg body weight/day, or approximately 75–100g daily, the total nitrogen and amino acid intake is sufficient to support the needs of all exercises. On this basis, the usual diet, supplying approximately 15–17% of the total energy as protein, should be adequate."

Still, this broad-brush approach to evaluating supplementation may overlook the benefits of taking certain vitamins, minerals, and amino acids in preparation for a marathon event. Although we agree that one gram of protein for each kilogram of body weight is sufficient in an athlete's diet, for example, we also believe that marathon runners can enhance performance by supplementing some of the amino acids beyond the usual levels.

Optimizing Your Performance

What follows is a supplementation program that can serve as a *guideline* for the long-distance runner. Dr. Roger Kendall, an associate professor of chemistry at Ambassador College who has specialized in the nutritional requirements of athletes, recommends the types of nutrients and dosages an endurance athlete can use to improve overall performance. He also explains the rationale and benefits of supplementing each of these nutrients.

Keep in mind, however, that this is not a one-size-fits-all plan. According to Dr. Kendall, the individual athlete should try various combinations of these nutrients and then monitor his or her performance to determine which supplements work best and in what size dosages. The point is to use the nutrient when it's needed most, perhaps throughout the training period or on the race day alone. When you reduce your aerobic effort, you also can reduce or eliminate your intake of these supplements.

The program focuses largely on the use of amino acids to improve long-distance running performance. As the building blocks of protein, amino acids play a big role in your energy production, muscle mass buildup, and fat-burning capability. The basic idea is to optimize the body's use of carbohydrates and fats during the long-distance event and limit its need to dip into the protein stored in muscles to fuel your performance. The more energy it has to derive from protein, the more it is stripping your body of the power needed to complete the event successfully.

In addition to amino acids, the endurance athlete may benefit from a multiple vitamin/mineral supplement, large doses of Vitamin C, and extra quantities of chromium, a mineral that affects the body's insulin production and its utilization of fat. In short, all of the nutrients discussed here reinforce the cardiovascular, circulatory, and immune systems, each of which plays a critical role in a marathon runner's performance.

Vitamins and Minerals

Multi-supplement

A good supplementation program starts with a moderately high-potency vitamin/mineral/amino acid multi-supplement. The multiple will serve as a foundation for any other supplements you take, preventing the imbalances that could occur if you take high dosages of isolated nutrients. As Dr. Kendall notes, all of these nutrients interact and work as a team in the body. Therefore, the task of improving your performance via supplementation will be difficult to accomplish if some of the team members are missing.

With a piecemeal approach to supplementation, you could help yourself in one area but harm yourself in another. Consider, for example, the athlete who takes megadoses of Vitamin C without adding calcium and magnesium to compensate for the increased amount of Vitamin C in the body. The most likely scenario is that about 80 percent of the Vitamin C would be eliminated from the body. In the process, it would carry away some quantities of calcium, magnesium, and other essential trace minerals that the body needs.

The athlete's need for additional vitamins has been explored in a number of studies over the years. One of the earliest of these was conducted by Dr. Roe at Cornell University in 1980. She demonstrated that female endurance athletes need at least twice the level of riboflavin, or Vitamin B_2, as more sedentary people. Although the study was limited to a specific group, it did show that athletes may require a vitamin intake in excess of the RDA. Another study conducted by Dr. McNeil at the University of Idaho demonstrated with an animal model that the conversion of carbohydrates (i.e., glucose) into energy required more thiamine, or Vitamin B_1.

The benefits of using a high-multiple vitamin/mineral supplement were demonstrated in a six-month study of marathoners conducted by Dr. Colden in Australia. In this study of twenty marathon runners, ten test subjects took a multiple-vitamin/mineral supplement while the other ten athletes served as control subjects. The study was done in a crossover fashion so that the researchers could track the effects of switching from a placebo to the multiple supplement.

The runners who took the supplement benefited in several significant ways. First, they achieved performance improvements by lowering their race times. They also improved their circulatory systems by reducing triglyceride and cholesterol levels. There was an 81 percent reduction in illness in the six-month period for those who took the supplement. And finally, the group had a better retention of glycogen and better muscle-mass retention.

Although critics of the study say that the groups weren't large enough to be statistically valid, this response shows that many people in the health field continue to criticize supplementation and nutritional intervention despite the evidence of its benefits, says Dr. Kendall. As a result, each runner will have to examine the available evidence and decide which approach is best for him- or herself.

Vitamin C

The traditional view of supplementation maintains that athletes do not benefit from doses of Vitamin C in excess of the RDA. In *Nutrition, Weight Control & Exercise* by Frank J. Katch and William D. McArdle, for example, the authors draw this conclusion about the vitamin's relationship to exercise: "While there is some indication that the Vitamin C requirement is increased in humans in times of stress, it has yet to be demonstrated that an excess of this vitamin is needed during physical training."

In our experience with runners, however, we have seen time and again that large doses of Vitamin C can help to prevent the muscle cramps and stiffness that occur following the completion of a long-distance race. Vitamin C serves as a key anti-stress and anti-fatigue nutrient. It is particularly important for collagen synthesis in long-distance runners, who break down tissue during the course of training and competing. Long-distance training also challenges the immune system, and Vitamin C can boost your immunity.

Although the RDA for Vitamin C is about 45 milligrams per day, endurance athletes can take anywhere from 2 to 10 grams daily of an ascorbate, chelated form of Vitamin C that includes key minerals, such as calcium, magnesium, manganese, and zinc. (Do not get the free form of ascorbic acid.) You may want to start by taking 1,000 milligrams of Vitamin C per day during the first week of training, and then add 1,000 milligrams at a time until you have reached what you believe to be your ideal level. On days that you have long training runs and on race day itself, you may take anywhere from 1,000 to 10,000 milligrams to help speed up the body's recovery process.

Chromium

In the past few years, research on GTF (glucose tolerance factor) chromium has shown that weight lifters and endurance athletes such as long-distance runners can achieve significant improvements with supplements of this essential nutrient. The use of GTF chromium, particularly the picinolate form at 200 micrograms twice daily, has substantial effects on the utilization of insulin and the burning of carbohydrates and fat. Indeed, the body's insulin mechanism cannot function properly without chromium.

Athletes may have a specific need for additional chromium. During an endurance event, their bodies will excrete two to three times the amount of chromium as that of the average sedentary individual. Not only must this lost chromium be replaced, but even more must be added to account for the additional calories you consume in preparation for the race. The supplemented GTF chromium will potentiate the body's insulin production, which, in turn, potentiates the uptake of glucose into the light tissues. This is where the glucose is converted to ATP, the energy molecule of the body.

GTF chromium's effect on insulin demonstrates the synergistic way in which the body works. As more glucose is transported to the tissues, you essentially achieve a better and more complete combustion of your carbohydrates. That means you will have a glycogen-sparing effect and a muscle-sparing effect. Rather than burn off the valuable protein in your muscles, your body will utilize the carbohydrates that are being stored as glycogen.

In addition, the increased production of insulin will increase the transport of the amino acids (discussed below) into the muscles. When you take GTF chromium, any amino acids you supplement will be taken up by the muscles due to the higher insulin activity. This restores energy to your muscles, which contributes to your stamina and endurance and enhances your ability to burn fat sources.

The RDA for chromium is 200 micrograms, but Dr. Kendall recommends that long-distance runners consider taking twice that much—or 400 micrograms—during the training period. Take one tablet in the morning and one at night. On race day, when you are using carbohydrate loading or similar techniques, you could take 600 micrograms.

Amino Acids

This supplementation program should help you to get optimum energy from carbohydrates and fats, thereby minimizing your body's use of protein stores as energy during the endurance event. If the body must burn off amino acids to produce energy, it is depleting muscle—the very storehouse in which you generate the power that propels you forward.

The amino acids described here have proven to be particularly important in the body's production and use of energy. To start, however, you should take a supplement that provides a complement of all twenty-two recognized amino acids, including both the "nonessential" amino acids (which are synthesized in the body) and the "essential" amino acids (which must be obtained from food). With this as a base, the additional doses of specific amino acids will not throw the system out of balance. A quality protein powder will do fine as a supplement.

This amino acid plays a central role in carbohydrate, fat, and protein metabolism. Research is showing that it improves aerobic performance by increasing energy output and oxygen utilization, by reducing the buildup of lactic acid in the muscles, and by improving the functioning of the immune system. Although the body makes DMG (i.e., it is nonessential) and food provides low levels of it, athletes who want to maximize their performance may want to take dosages that exceed the RDA.

DMG was first appreciated as Vitamin B_{15} about ten years ago. The Russians studied the amino acid and found that it was very beneficial during sports practice. It improved energy output and performance and reduced lactic-acid buildup. Dr. Kendall's own research has also shown that DMG reduces lactic-acid buildup during aerobic activity. This is a significant benefit, because many runners suffer from cramping and pain as lactic acid builds in the bloodstream and eventually the muscle tissue. Long-distance runners produce lactic acid as their supply of oxygen is depleted. The body's ability to use the available oxygen goes down as the carbon dioxide goes up.

The beneficial effects of DMG were first noted in race horses. Although many horses can achieve a strong performance during the first three-quarters of a mile, they completely peter out at the end of the race. When these animals took DMG, however, they could take 1.5 seconds off their race time. The difference was significant enough to start turning losers into winners. As a result, more and more trainers have added DMG to their training programs.

Animal research also has demonstrated that DMG reduces the lactic-acid buildup caused by emotional or mental stress, says Dr. Kendall. When the muscles are not even moving, the "anxiety syndrome" can cause glycogen stores to be depleted, oxygen to be consumed, and lactic acid to be produced. But this chain of events did not occur when animals were given DMG, and no lactic acid was produced. Other studies have shown that the energy output is increased with DMG supplements. The results are significant, considering that the average reduction in lactic-acid buildup was 30 to 40 percent in several of the studies.

DMG also can enhance your performance by strengthening the immune system, which often suffers from the physical, mental, and emotional stress produced by endurance training. In many cases, athletes who train too hard not only become fatigued but also get more colds, cold sores, and viral infections. They may discover that it takes them longer to recover as well. DMG supplements can help those athletes significantly.

The following dosages of DMG are recommended for the day of an endurance event lasting for three to five hours. Keep in mind, however, that an individual's need could vary in either direction. Some may need more, some less. But all runners can significantly increase the current recommended level of 300 to 400 milligrams. Thirty minutes before the race, take four 125 milligram tablets (500 milligrams total). During the race, as you deplete your glycogen stores, take two more tablets every four miles to prevent pain and stiffness.

Carnitine

This amino acid is vital to the process of burning fatty acids. Carnitine is the biochemical transporter of fatty acids across the membrane of the mitochondria, which is the energy factory within the muscle cell that breaks down glucose into ATP, the energy molecule of the body. In essence, the body inter-converts the fatty acids into carbohydrates and then burns them off. The increased ability to burn fat leads to better muscle development, as well as a glycogen-sparing effect if your fatty acid metabolism is impaired.

Carnitine supplements may be especially important for vegetarians because the amino acid is only found in animal foodstuffs. Although it can also be produced in the body, you must have adequate levels of lysine, methionine, Vitamin C, niacin, and Vitamin B_1 in order to do so. Hence, Dr. Kendall believes a better approach is to supplement carnitine as part of the training program to optimize your fat-burning capability. Several studies are being conducted in Italy now, he says, to examine the effects of carnitine on the glycogen storage, total energy output, and fat-burning mechanism of long-distance runners and cyclists.

Be aware that two types of this amino acid, L-carnitine and

D-carnitine, may be available at health-food stores. L-carnitine provides the benefits described here, whereas D-carnitine has been shown to cause some health problems. According to Dr. Kendall, athletes may consider taking 250 milligrams of L-carnitine three times daily during training, or a total of 750 milligrams. On race day, they can take slightly more.

One word of caution, however: The sale of carnitine as an over-the-counter food supplement has caused some concern in medical circles. In the *Townsend Letter for Doctors* (November 1991), an executive of Sigma-Tau Pharmaceuticals Inc., which makes a carnitine product sold by prescription only, warns that the indiscriminate and unsupervised use of L-carnitine poses a potential risk for individuals who have glucose regulatory abnormalities and undiagnosed metabolic disorders.

The crux of the problem, says this executive, is that L-carnitine potentially may "alter the complex fuel substrate flux in patients with glucose regulatory abnormalities and thereby cause hyperglycemia or hypoglycemia with the inherent clinical risks associated with these conditions." Likewise, he warns that the L-carnitine food supplement may be used by people with metabolic disorders without a diagnosis of the underlying problem and the benefit of a doctor's supervision.

Free-Form Amino Acids

Research is now demonstrating that specific amino acids can improve performance. During an endurance event, the muscles are constantly being worked and torn down. The body throws out the waste products and continues to build up the protein that goes into the muscle fibers. If you get this protein from food, however, the digestive system must break down the protein and assimilate the individual amino acids that it will utilize.

As stated earlier, a better way to restore the muscle mass that's lost during an aerobic event is to take a product that contains the amino acids before the workout begins. In addition, the following amino acids deserve special consideration:

▶ Arginine and Lysine: These two amino acids have been researched because of their impact on the human growth

181

hormone, which helps to reduce body fat and increase muscle mass. Research conducted in Italy has shown that a better muscle-mass retention can be achieved with one gram each of arginine and lysine.

Dr. Kendall believes that these amino acids may have an impact on the insulin response. Insulin, the growth hormone, and testosterone are potent anabolic hormones. Insulin plays an important role in the transport and utilization of carbohydrates (glucose), and it facilitates the uptake of protein by the muscles. The anabolic effects will occur when you have adequate insulin levels present in the body, and this may be the function that arginine and lysine play in aerobic performance.

A small amount of arginine and lysine, in the 100-milligram range, will do little to enhance performance. In general, says Dr. Kendall, the studies show that two grams of arginine and lysine (in a 1-to-1 blend) should be taken at least once a day. Some athletes may want to take these amino acids on race day only, rather than throughout the training period.

▶ Branched-Chain Amino Acids (BCAAs): More than 20 percent of all energy derived in the muscles comes from these three amino acids, which include leucine, isoleucine, and valine. Again, these amino acids will help your body to burn fat and spare the protein during endurance training. As a result, your energy needs will be better balanced and your muscle-mass retention will be improved. The increased fat-burning capability is especially important because the heart, as a muscle, derives it energy from fat rather than from carbohydrates.

Dr. Kendall recommends that an athlete take the BCAAs along with arginine, lysine, and the other free form amino acids to prevent the body from becoming unbalanced by high levels of a single amino acid. Many athletes have taken a blend of just one to two grams of the BCAAs, says Dr. Kendall, and have reported in an anecdotal fashion that their workouts improved as a result.

Special Supplements

In addition to the basics—vitamins, minerals, and amino acids—marathon runners may want to supplement coenzyme Q and primrose oil.

Coenzyme Q

This co-factor is involved in the electron transfer process that takes place when you burn carbohydrates and produce the high-energy ATP molecules. Because coenzyme Q is an electron receptor, your energy capacity will be reduced when it is in short supply. Again, the body can produce coenzyme Q if the right amino acids, accessory co-factors, vitamins, and minerals are in place, but the endurance athlete would do better to supplement it as part of a dietary program.

Coenzyme Q was first discovered and used in Japan, which has produced a number of nutritional and therapeutic advances in the field of clinical nutrition. Although there have not been many studies to date that looked at specific performance gains, coenzyme Q has been found to potentiate the immune system, improve oxygen utilization, and serve as an antioxidant.

Much like the other nutrients discussed here, coenzyme Q will help to optimize the production of energy, enhance the immune system, and trigger the body's antioxidant effects, which help to depollute the body by deactivating or neutralizing the free radicals that destroy cell membranes and enzymes that are involved in the energy process. Coenzyme Q also can improve wound healing. From a therapeutic point of view, it has been used in congestive heart failure and rheumatic heart conditions that signal a deficiency of circulation within the heart.

The body's own ability to produce coenzyme Q will lessen with age. Therefore, this supplement may not be as important for a twenty-year-old runner as it is for the forty-year-old endurance athlete who wants to improve his or her race time. In the latter case, some additional coenzyme Q10, which has been called the "spark plug" of the energy production within the mitochondria, can provide the needed boost. The therapeutic dosages of coenzyme Q10 now range from 30 to 100 milligrams. Dr. Kendall recommends that an athlete take from 25 to 50 milligrams on race day.

Primrose Oil

Supplements of the essential fatty acids, especially primrose oil, may be needed by some long-distance runners, such as postmenopausal women. The GLA (Gamma Linonenic Acid) variety will counter the negative effects of reduced estrogen in the body and, in essence, provide a hormonal effect. Other men and women may find that they are deficient in essential fatty acids due to stress and other factors. These fatty acids are important because they tend to control some of the free radical processes taking place in the body, such as inflammation. Therefore, athletes can take a 500-milligram capsule of primrose oil six times a day, or 3 grams total, both during training and on race day.

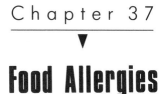

Chapter 37
▼
Food Allergies

People who are allergic to certain foods and substances can suffer from many health problems, including a reduction in their energy levels. These people live with a highly sensitive condition that stems from a wide variety of causes and leads to an equally broad range of symptoms. As an ancient poet and philosopher once said, "One man's meat is another man's poison."

The body designs the allergic mechanism to protect itself from an allergen that the cells perceive to be a foreign substance. In essence, the cells overreact to the presence of the "invader." This hypersensitivity can produce reactions so complex and varied that many people who have food or environmental allergies are labeled hypochondriacs. These people often are unaware of the underlying cause of their illness. And most practicing physicians and allergists also are in the dark when it comes to identifying the true root of the problems.

Allergies cause a state of distress in millions of people who suffer on a daily basis. Some allergists and environmental medicine experts estimate that roughly 15 percent of the population has at least one allergy that is serious enough to require medical attention. The general population is most sensitive to the foods that are eaten most frequently. These include milk, wheat, yeast, corn, eggs, beef, sugar, citrus fruits, potatoes, tomatoes, and coffee.

People who are sensitive to foods, chemicals, or other environmental allergens may experience any of the following common symptoms: insomnia, headache, fatigue, rapid mood swings, confusion, depression, anxiety, hyperactivity, heart palpitations, muscle aches and joint pains, bed-wetting, rhinitis, uticaria (hives), shortness of breath, diarrhea, and constipation. The reaction may occur immediately following exposure to an allergen, such as when a person feels drowsy after a meal, or it may be delayed for several hours after the initial contact.

The symptoms are diversified because any organ system in the body can react to an allergen. A cerebral response may cause paranoia or depression, for example, while a gastrointestinal response causes bloating, diarrhea, or constipation. Different foods can even cause different reactions in the same individual. If a person has a cerebral allergy to wheat and a gastrointestinal sensitivity to milk, he or she may experience both fatigue and irritable bowel syndrome from a breakfast of whole-wheat toast and milk. The different organ symptoms can respond negatively to the two foods.

Causes of Hypersensitivity

Why do people become sensitive to their environment? According to the "allergy threshold concept," a culmination of factors will cause a person to cross the threshold and become allergic to certain substances. These include external factors, such as environmental pollutants and the weather, as well as internal factors, such as genetic makeup, stress, nutritional deficiencies, immune status, and age. Psychological and emotional stress, for example, can be strong enough to trigger an allergic response. In some cases, stress can even cause the allergy.

Heredity plays a primary role in the development of allergies. When both parents have allergies, their children have a 75 percent chance of inheriting a predisposition to the condition. When one parent has an allergy, the chance is 50 percent. The child does not have to inherit the same allergic response, however. The mother may be allergic to wheat, whereas the child is allergic to milk. The mother may have asthma, whereas the child has eczema. In other cases, babies can develop allergies to the same foods as the mother through the placenta, while in the womb, or through breast-feeding after birth.

Allergies also may result from nutritional deficiencies and biochemical and hormonal imbalances. These deficiencies can be caused by eating a limited variety of foods, eating too many foods that are high in refined carbohydrates, or smoking cigarettes. Indeed, it is usually a combination of many factors that causes a person to become hypersensitive.

Finally, an impaired digestive system underlies most food allergies. To digest food properly, the body must secrete hydrochloric acid into the stomach along with pancreatic enzymes. These substances break down the large protein molecules into small molecules for absorption and utilization. If the digestive system is impaired, however, it may not secrete enough digestive juices or enzymes. The large molecules will go directly into the bloodstream. This can cause an allergy because the immune system reacts to the molecules as if they were foreign invaders. As a result, the person now has an allergic response to the food that the body could not break down.

To alleviate these allergies, the person must correct any nutritional deficiencies and digestive imbalances. In addition, any stress that leads a person to the allergic threshold must be eliminated or reduced, whether they be caused by environmental factors or internal factors. The healthier our physical and mental environment, the better we can achieve and maintain a state of well-being.

Types of Food Allergies

People can develop several types of food allergies, including a cyclic allergy, a fixed allergy, and an addictive allergic reaction.

► Cyclic allergies: This type of allergy, the most common form, occurs when a person eats the offending foods frequently and the effects become cumulative. If the food is discontinued and the exposure is reduced (no more than once in five days), the food can be tolerated again in small amounts. Therefore, people with cyclic allergies can remain symptom-free if they eat the foods on an infrequent basis.

Other factors can influence the degree of sensitivity, however. These include infection, emotional stress, fatigue, overeating, the condition of the food (fresh, raw, cooked, etc.), the presence of pollution and other environmental allergens, and a change in temperature. The accumulation of these adverse factors will determine whether a person becomes symptomatic.

To change these allergies, all of the negative factors must be addressed. Generally, it's not enough to stop eating the food. You must improve your nutritional status, avoid any chemical and inhalant offenders, and reduce emotional stress. You also have to pay more attention to food combinations. You may be able to tolerate a food by itself, for example, that will cause an allergic reaction when it is mixed with other foods in the same meal. The duration and severity of the resulting symptoms depend largely upon how long the allergens remain in the body. As a result, constipation can extend the body's reaction to an allergen.

► Fixed allergies: This sensitivity causes you to react to a certain type of food every time you eat it. No matter how long you have abstained from eating the food or how little you have eaten, the allergic response takes place. A person who is allergic to strawberries, for example, may get hives on his or her face every time he or she eats a fresh strawberry or strawberry jam. A physician can usually detect these allergens through testing procedures or a comprehensive case history.

► Addictive allergic response: With this type of allergy, you crave the foods to which you are allergic. These cravings can lead to an addictive state. Consequently, low-grade, chronic symptoms often accompany this type of allergy, and withdrawal symptoms occur when the food is not eaten. To lessen the symptoms, you eat some form of the very foods that have initiated the underlying problems.

This allergic response often remains hidden or masked because you do not suspect the foods that alleviate your symptoms as the real culprit. In fact, you will typically feel better right after you eat the foods. That will make it difficult for you and your physician to pinpoint the offending food, particularly if the doctor is not properly trained in treating allergies.

The process of treating allergies is complicated by the fact that the different types do not always occur along the clear-cut lines described above. If a fixed allergy during infancy is not recognized, for example, it can become an addictive allergic reaction later in life. This often happens with commonly eaten foods, such as milk, which we believe to be essential for all people. When a baby is allergic to milk, he or she may have an acute reaction, such as breaking out in hives or spitting up. If the parents do not recognize this as an allergic reaction and continue to give the child milk, he or she may develop more general and less obvious types of symptoms. In essence, the body attempts to adapt to the acute reaction, eventually producing chronic symptoms, such as arthritis, fatigue, depression, or headaches.

Environmental Medicine

Unlike traditional branches of medicine, which often treat allergies and other problems with drugs and surgery, environmental medicine offers alternative treatments that are less invasive. Its practitioners apply the principles of holistic medicine to care for the whole being as an integral part of the ecosystem.

Experts in environmental medicine can properly treat the problems that arise from food, chemical, and inhalant allergies. Their understanding of allergies extends far beyond the typical reactions, such as a runny nose, watery eyes, rash, hay fever, hives, or asthma.

The field of environmental medicine has developed diagnostic and therapeutic programs that represent the first comprehensive medical effort to trace the negative effects that we have suffered while moving from a relatively simple, largely rural existence to a complex, industrial, and predominantly urban society. As such, this branch of medicine is challenging modern medicine's narrow view of allergies and diseases. It should gain even more attention in the coming years as the public continues to lose faith in traditional medicine, which clearly cannot cure many of our common illnesses.

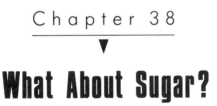

Chapter 38

▼

What About Sugar?

Many athletes mistakenly rely on sugar for energy and a "lift." But contrary to popular belief, the typical coffee and doughnut break actually worsens fatigue and stresses the vital organs by sending too much glucose into the bloodstream. Although you do need carbohydrates to supply energy, and especially to fuel your brain, you don't need to add processed sugar to your diet at all. When you eat a well-balanced diet that contains complex carbohydrates and promotes healthy metabolism, the liver will supply any energy needed by the working muscles from its reserves.

Our society's addiction to sugar has had a serious impact on cardiovascular well-being. As our sugar intake has risen dramatically, so has the incidence of heart disease. Sugar compounds the damage that too much fat can cause in the body. Eating sugar probably prompts the liver to produce excess fats, which then circulate in the blood. Sugar may cause such disorders as ulcers or Type IV hyperlipidemia, which may then lead to diabetes and other serious conditions. Animal studies also have shown that sugar (especially sucrose) can damage major organs, veins, and arteries and increase the buildup of plaque in the arteries. When rodents are fed sugar, especially when they are young, their lives are shortened.

As an athlete, you should learn to recognize the types of sugar that various foods contain and eliminate them from your diet. As described here, the consequences of a life-long sugar habit can be serious indeed.

Types of Sugar

All forms of refined sugar, including sucrose (cane sugar), glucose (corn sugar), and fructose (honey sugar), tend to raise the triglyceride and cholesterol levels in the blood, two factors that contribute to cardiovascular disease. Although some people consider the fructose in fruits and honey to be a superior form of sugar, its real advantage lies in the fact that it is sweeter than glucose and sucrose (whose molecule is half fructose and half glucose). The fructose-rich honey is sweeter than table sugar and much sweeter than corn syrup.

The inexpensive, refined sugar used in large quantities in packaged foods may go by the name of glucose, corn syrup, corn sugar, or dextrose. More than one of these may be deceptively listed on the labels of carbohydrate foods, along with sugar, honey, sucrose, maltose, and lactose. Refined sugar most likely is the main ingredient of a product that contains more than one of these sugars, even if they are not listed first on the label. Remember, too, that pure glucose has the same effect on metabolism as other refined sugars, even though it does not taste very sweet.

When many people think of sugar's harmful effects, tooth decay and extra pounds naturally come to mind. But its potential damage is much more extensive, according to Dr. John Yudkin, one of the world's leading authorities on sugar in the diet. Sugar can produce the following effects in the body: irregularities in the insulin response; diabetes-like damage to the kidneys; degeneration of the retina; higher blood fat levels; and increasing stickiness of the blood platelets, a common precursor of heart trouble.

The traditional medical establishment tends to ignore the link between sugar and disease. But even the more conventional epidemiology studies have shown that the more sugar in the diet, the greater the chances that cardiac trouble will develop in certain people or worsen in those who already suffer from a heart condition. Unrefined carbohydrates and fiber are safer than processed carbohydrates and help to protect the heart, liver, and other vital organs.

According to recent research, the following conditions may be caused or complicated by sugar: elevated triglyceride and cholesterol level, especially in middle-aged men and menopausal women, ulcers, hyperlipidemia, high blood pressure, myocardial infarction, and ischemic heart disease. Animal studies show that high-sugar diets are responsible in part for the fatty degeneration of the inner coat of the arteries.

People who suffer from hypertension have learned to avoid salt in their diets. But they may not know that sugar can harm the kidneys and heart, too. Animal studies suggest that high blood pressure may lead to blood sugar disorders. Therefore, those with hypertension have even more reason to eliminate sugar from their diet.

Too much refined sugar and flour in the diet may lead to hypoglycemia, or low blood sugar, which reduces the supply of glucose needed by the brain "circuits" to communicate properly. This condition can distort a person's perceptions, emotions, and behavior. Indeed, too much refined sugar may negatively affect people's behavior in the following ways: Children may become hyperkinetic or learning-disabled, young people may become learning-disabled or delinquent, and adults may behave criminally.

This observation has been verified by studies and the clinical experience of educators, psychologists, parents, and probation and prison officials. As a result, some institutions now refuse to order refined sugar and flour products. They include the Los Angeles County Probation Department, the Los Angeles and New York City school systems, and the Naval Correctional Center in Seattle.

The millions of Americans who suffer from hypoglycemia should not take the condition lightly. It can cause relatively minor problems, such as too much snacking and napping due to the hunger and fatigue it causes, but it can also lead to severe disorders, such as diabetes and schizophrenia. If you continue to eat a diet that's high in refined carbohydrates, especially sugar, you are inviting damage to your brain and nervous system. Neither can survive without a constant supply of glucose in the bloodstream. Consequently, hypoglycemics should eliminate stimulants such as sugar, caffeine, and cigarettes and develop a healthy diet that emphasizes protein. A nutritionist can recommend any supplements you may need.

Those who eliminate refined sugar from their diets will have a greater resistance to infections as well. All forms of sugar, particularly sucrose, depress the protective functions of the cells. A lower sugar content in your meals also helps to maintain normal levels of acid and pepsin in the stomach. And finally, the elimination of refined sugar often results in visible healing of skin conditions such as acne.

A Final Word

It should be noted that even natural sugar can pose problems for some people. If they are sensitive to the lactose or milk sugar in dairy products, for example, they may suffer from gastrointestinal problems such as primary, secondary, or temporary malabsorption of the lactose.

Clearly, there are good reasons for all of us to reduce our sugar intake. People with good health habits—exercising, keeping their weight normal, and not smoking—are ahead of the game in avoiding the killer diseases. But for even greater protection, they should switch from sugary pick-me-ups to complex carbohydrates that are rich in fiber. Snacks such as whole-grain crackers, popcorn, and raw fruits will reduce cholesterol, maintain a normal amount of blood fats, and keep the entire body healthy.

Chapter 39
▼

What About Fiber?

In recent years, bread and cereal manufacturers have awakened to the fact that fiber plays an essential role in promoting intestinal health. Unfortunately, their response has been to charge us extra to add fiber to the very products from which they have been removing it for decades. A variety of foods include natural fiber, however, so you don't have to pay that price to get the roughage you need.

The cell walls of all fruits, vegetables, seeds, nuts, and grains contain the ingredients of fiber, including cellulose, hemicellulose, pectin, lignin, and several gums. These complex polysaccharides, known collectively as fiber, give plants the ability to grow up structurally strong.

Fiber is vital to our body functioning as well, even though it is nondigestible. Fibers form a special group of carbohydrates that provide a kind of janitorial service for our intestines by keeping them free of hazardous substance, including powerful carcinogens. Refined carbohydrates and protein foods such as milk, cheese, and beef cannot do this job.

The Need for Fiber

Although fiber cannot be digested and used nutritionally, it provides the roughage needed to clean the entire intestinal tract and keep it free of a wide variety of poisonous substances. Fiber also scrubs the cell walls of the colon and bowels, hastening the time that it takes foods to travel through the digestive system. Consequently, the body will not hold toxins any longer than it must.

A high-fiber diet leads to a generous supply of friendly bacteria in the colon. These microorganisms, which partially fragment most fibers, proliferate when you eat a diet that's rich in natural carbohydrate fiber. Conversely, if your diet is high in fatty meats, no-fiber breads, and sugary desserts, fewer of these disease-preventing organisms will be present in the intestinal tract. With a low-fiber diet, their normal food supply is absent, and they are not needed.

People who do not eat an adequate supply of fiber may be at risk for constipation, colorectal cancer, or other common diseases of the gastrointestinal system. This risk increases when a diet is high in fat and sugar but low in fresh, nutritious, and wholesome foods. Inactivity creates even more stress in this situation. You should be checked for colorectal cancer during your annual physical examination. Report any signs of the disease to your doctor immediately.

To keep your bowels healthy and protect against certain types of cancer, your diet should include a high intake of natural fiber foods, moderate amounts of protein, and a low fat intake. Indeed, vegetarians who eat a high-fiber, low-fat diet run the least risk of developing these diseases.

Fiber foods provide several other benefits as well. They stimulate and exercise the mouth, gums, oral membranes, and facial muscles, for example. Fiber also encourages appetite control because it absorbs fluid and creates the satisfied feeling you crave when dieting. For the most part, however, fiber does not contribute too many calories. And when you feel full, you won't be tempted to snack too much.

Fiber Requirements

For healthy people, 10 to 12 grams daily of natural fiber should be an adequate supply. Those who suffer from pressure diseases or occasional bouts of irregularity may need extra amounts. In the latter case, for example, you could sprinkle a few extra teaspoons of an untreated, unheated fiber product on your morning cereal or evening salad. Try wheat germ, wheat bran, or even rice or corn bran for some variety.

You may prefer to use salad foods and fruits to meet your roughage requirements. In that case, have a raw salad for lunch, a partially cooked salad such as tabouli for dinner, and a big puree of fresh fruit in season. These foods would meet the body's needs quite well, but you should be aware that some researchers believe that they absorb the most amount of water in your intestines.

Grain Sources

Fiber foods such as grains, should be eaten in their natural form. Our bodies, which have evolved from our ancestors' eating habits, can absorb a food's total value, including vitamins, minerals, trace minerals, enzymes, and the bulk needed for bowel movements. It's worth the extra minutes that it takes to cook grains from scratch. Whole-wheat breads and unprocessed cereals—the real things—can be bought at a natural-foods store.

Remember that unrefined, whole grains are triple-layered foods. Each of these layers is packed with nutrients. The first layer is bran. The second is the endosperm, which is rich in starch and protein. And at the heart of the grain is the germ, which contains protein, essential fats, and Vitamins B and E.

Bran, in particular, has become a popular source of fiber. While it's fine to eat some bran every day to improve your health and regulate your bowel movements, be sure to include it as part of a well-balanced diet. The fiber in fruits and vegetables provides different values than the fiber in grains. Your goal should be to eat a variety of foods that offer many nutrients, including various sources of fiber.

Most store-bought breads and cereals have the germ and bran removed. Although some brands are later "fortified" to compensate for that removal, it's not the same as eating natural whole foods. Cereal manufacturers have processed their supermarket brands according to profit motives and the belief that fiber served no useful purpose. Now that we know better, processing methods are slowly changing, and supermarkets are carrying some whole-fiber breakfast cereals.

Some of these "natural" cereals are deceptive, however. Read the label carefully to determine that it is a whole-grain product and that it does not contain large amounts of sugar and preservatives. Why pay more for devitalized foods that have been processed an extra step to return what was taken out? The more food is treated, heated, and handled during processing, the more its value declines. When in doubt, stick with old favorites, such as non-instant oatmeal, cracked wheat, undergerminated corn meal, brown rice, and buckwheat groats (kasha).

Fruit and Vegetable Sources

Buy fresh fruits and vegetables in season and eat them raw whenever possible. One easy way to eat raw vegetables is to grate them in a salad. In other cases, you can cook them in as little water as possible to protect the nutrients. Use "waterless" cookware or an inexpensive steamer that slips into a saucepan. Avoid both frozen and canned vegetables, which are a poor second to fresh foods. If you must eat them on occasion, however, frozen foods are the better choice. They retain more nutrients and fiber and contain less sodium.

Not all vegetables contain an equal amount of fiber, of course. Heading the list are many of the root vegetables, whose crunchy quality and hardness provide a high-fiber yield. Because your whole mouth must be used to eat these vegetables, they also give your jaws and teeth a beneficial workout. Be sure to eat the vegetable skin as well. Much of a plant's roughage and nutrients are stored in and near the skin. The less common tubers, such as yams, kohlrabi, parsnips, and eggplants, also can be eaten whole.

Don't neglect the legume family when it comes to obtaining fiber. You can eat peas, chick peas, mung beans, and lentils—skin and all—by sprouting them instead of cooking them. That way, you'll get the full value of the live food, including amino acids, minerals, and carbohydrate energy.

Protopectin

Among the fruit family, grapefruits and oranges deserve special consideration. The pulp of all citrus fruit contains a two-carbohydrate food factor called protopectin. This combination of cellulose and pectin has generated considerable interest in the biochemistry field. Even vegetables are an occasional secondary source of these nutrients.

You benefit from both ingredients: The cellulose absorbs fluid from your intestines and begins to enlarge, quickly pushing along the contents of the digestive tract. The pectin, meanwhile, becomes gelatinous and balances the actions of the cellulose by providing lubrication and smooth passage for the food. Protopectin also helps your body to get the most value from other nutritious foods and to use dietary fats in a better way. This protects you from the cardiovascular dangers of a high cholesterol count.

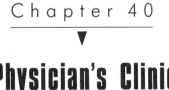

Chapter 40

▼

A Physician's Clinical Perspective

How strong is the link between nutrition and athletic performance? To answer that vital question, we went to the New

York offices of Dr. Christopher Calapai, a physician who advises athletes and others on nutrition and preventive health.

Like Dr. Kendall, a research scientist (see Chapter 36), Dr. Calapai suggests that athletes may need to supplement specific nutrients in their diets, based on individual needs. Although the two doctors come from different perspectives—one's a researcher and one's a practicing clinician—their conclusions about the need for supplementation are much the same.

Here's what Dr. Calapai had to say about the importance of proper nutrition in athletic endeavors and the need to identify and address any roadblocks to optimal health. Included are case studies of patients who have overcome their own nutritional obstacles by addressing fundamental problems in their diets.

Once you are committed to an athletic regimen, maximizing your nutritional state may be the most important step you take. In the pursuit of health, an athlete desperately needs to meet his or her nutritional requirements, supplying the body with the substances that stimulate immune function, increase aerobic capacity, produce energy, and enhance cardiovascular fitness.

Vitamins and minerals play a critical role in maintaining health and treating various disorders. The body needs them for proper functioning of the muscles, nerves, skin, heart, lung, brain, and other organs and systems. What's more, deficiencies have been linked to everything from asthma, hypertension, and cardiovascular disease to chronic fatigue, immune dysfunction, and various cancers.

We are all individual in many ways, however, especially in our physiochemical makeup. Each person's nutrient requirements will depend on such factors as genetic makeup, age, sex, and activity level. Therefore, it's essential to have a nutritional protocol tailored to your specific needs.

Where does the process begin? Once you have defined your exercise goals—to improve strength, coordination, flexibility, or cardiovascular status and endurance—start by considering whether you face any barriers to exercise or have medical conditions that need to be addressed. These may include hypertension, obesity, atherosclerosis, diabetes, hypoglycemia, kidney or liver disease, asthma, and even cancer. Likewise, your exercise capacity can be affected by a physical or musculoskeletal problem, including short-leg and-arm syndromes, arthritis, and spinal disorders such as scoliosis and spinal bifida.

Any of these conditions can interfere with optimal functioning. Realistically, it is not a good idea to exercise when you are ill or feel run down. Exercise can be more damaging than beneficial if you are deficient in nutrients or suffer from heart disease, asthma, immune system dysfunction, or "burnout." A more prudent approach is to maximize your health status before you undertake demanding activities. You need to detoxify and rebuild the body to get the most benefits from exercise.

Pre-exercise Assessment

For athletes of any type, the first line of defense is to undergo a pre-exercise health and fitness assessment. This process will give you and your doctor a complete picture of your chemistry, physiology, and anatomy, as well as your nutritional, medical, and emotional makeup.

In fact, you may very well set yourself up for injury if you exercise without such an assessment. A classic example is the "weekend warrior" who suffers recurring injuries and illnesses because he or she does not exercise or eat properly during the week and then overexerts him- or herself during some weekend activity. These people are an orthopedic surgeon's dream, whether they be runners, skiers, ball players, or tennis and golf enthusiasts.

The pre-exercise assessment includes a variety of tests and evaluations, all of which add up to a "comprehensive approach to health care." With this approach, the focus is on finding and correcting the *cause* of an illness or disease, rather than on treating symptoms that may have as many as ten different causes. The comprehensive approach also puts the emphasis on learning about the whole person and then teaching that person about him- or herself. It's preventive medicine, aimed at achieving optimal health by maximizing nutrition and exercise.

The workup encompasses the following evaluations and testing procedures:

▶ Patient history. This category includes a number of subcomponents: personal and family medical history; allergies to foods, inhalants, or chemicals; the foods, beverages, and nutrients in the person's diet; surgical history; social factors such as smoking, alcohol, or drug abuse; any medications taken regularly and as needed; and an emotional/psychological stress analysis.

▶ Physical examination. This includes testing for strength, range of motion, coordination, and musculoskeletal function, along with an examination of all the body systems (including digestive, cardiovascular, neurological, skin, and others). A thorough physical exam determines the current level of functioning and reveals minor abnormalities that may be linked to previously undiscovered illnesses.

▶ Complete blood count (CBC). This test detects abnormalities in red and white blood cells that will affect body functioning. Anemia or a low red-blood cell count, for example, can decrease oxygen uptake and contribute to fatigue, a common condition in female athletes. The test also includes a look at immune functioning through neutrophils, eosinophils, and monocytes. In many cases, the monocyte count is elevated with viral syndrome.

▶ Chemistry. These tests measure the levels of blood sugar, thyroid function, cholesterol, triglyceride, HDL, and protein, as well as the digestive and absorptive capacity, liver and kidney function, and cardiac risk. The tests may reveal silent or asymptomatic diseases in many people, such as low or high blood sugar. Exercise can bring high sugar into a normal range and can even help prevent or lessen Type II or insulin-dependent diabetes. A chemistry assessment is equally essential for people with heart disease or circulatory disorders. In fact, it could be quite dangerous for these people to begin exercising without a thorough evaluation.

▶ Vitamin and mineral assays (Nutriscan). Everyone should

receive this assessment of the nutrient levels in the body, regardless of his or her health status. Without it, you have no way of knowing exactly what your body lacks. Recent research shows that deficiencies in various nutrients can put a person at high risk for disorders ranging from hypertension to heart disease and cancer. Low selenium, for example, has been linked to cardiomyopathy, a heart muscle disorder, while low magnesium can cause chronic fatigue, asthma, and hypertension. Meanwhile, low levels of Vitamins A, C, E, and beta carotene may be related to various cancers, heart disease, and cataracts.

► Urinalysis. This test, which evaluates the amount of protein, sugar, bacteria, and ketones in the urine, provides indirect information on kidney function, diabetes, and urinary tract infections. A 24-hour urine test assesses the amount of exposure to heavy metals. These factors are important because kidney function plays a vital role in exercising. As the intensity of exercise increases, so does the demand placed on the kidneys, which have to work harder to filter the blood.

► Electrocardiogram. An EKG evaluates the electrical function of the heart, specifically the rate and rhythm of the heartbeat. Many people have irregular beats when they are either resting or exercising, and this must be corrected before they can engage in strenuous activity.

► Halter monitor. This device provides a 24-hour reading of the heart. In doing so, it gives much more detailed information about the number of irregular, skipped, or dropped beats.

► Stress test. During this test, an EKG measures irregular heartbeats while you are physically stressed by walking on a treadmill. Anyone who engages in strenuous activity should consider taking the test, especially those over the age of thirty-five.

► Doppler/sonography. This simple, noninvasive procedure uses sound waves to produce a picture of the organs and vessels, thereby revealing any abnormal masses, tumors, or deposits of plaque on the blood-vessel walls.

▶ Height, weight, blood pressure, and pulse. These basic indicators also are important in evaluating health status.

▶ Viral titers. In recent years, more people have been suffering from viral syndromes, including Epstein-Barr virus, cytomegalo-virus, herpes, and even HIV. The increasing incidence of these syndromes may be due to their ease of transmission or to the poor functioning of many people's immune systems. In fact, nutrient deficiencies can hinder immune cell production and set the stage for a decreased ability to fight a virus or bacteria.

▶ Nutritional assessment. This category includes an evaluation of various factors: the frequency of eating (one, two, three, or more times a day); the quantity of food in the diet; the quality of foods being eaten, including proteins, carbohydrates, fats and oils, sugar, alcohol, preservatives, dyes, colorings, animal oils/fats, and liquids; the status of vitamins and minerals; a review of absorptive capacity; an analysis of body composition (by percentages of fat, lean muscle, and water); and an evaluation of the stool for fiber content, undigested fibers, consistency, bacteria or pathogens, yeast, and blood.

The Physiology of Exercise

It's important to recognize that exercise places significant demands on the body's metabolism. To start, the heart rate increases as you begin physical exercise. Obviously, this increases the circulation of blood, oxygen, and nutrients to all of the body tissues. As your muscles contract, you utilize minerals, such as calcium, magnesium, and potassium. That means that you must replenish the body with such minerals to sustain high levels of exercise.

The longer you exercise, the greater the amount of oxygen delivered to the tissues and the more you depend on oxygen for energy production. This is called aerobic metabolism. By contrast, anaerobic metabolism involves energy production without oxygen. This occurs in the first few minutes of exercise, before a large amount of oxygen can be taken in.

Some types of exercise increase strength, of course, while others improve cardiovascular fitness. To achieve optimal health and functioning, it's best to blend these activities so that you can maximize your fitness in every way, enhancing your strength, posture, coordination, stamina, and endurance.

Weight training, for example, will increase the size and strength of muscles but offers little cardiovascular benefit. Still, the training can improve your posture, walking or gait, balance, and physical performance in various sports. The weight training will "pump" the muscles full of blood that carries some oxygen and nutrients. When aerobic exercises are performed right after, you get a boost of oxygen to all the tissues that can enhance the metabolic effect of exercise.

To maximize aerobic benefits, you need to involve as much muscle mass as possible. Therefore, swimming is more beneficial for the heart than, say, stair climbing, because more muscles are being utilized and worked. One of the best, safest, and easiest types of aerobic activity is power walking, which involves many muscles but causes little or no undue stress to the tissues. Power walking, which can be done virtually anywhere and anytime, is the exercise for all ages.

Likewise, running is a great activity both aerobically and physically. It offers tremendous cardiovascular benefits, provided you design a running program that plots out a slow and gradual increase in intensity over a period of time. People who are out of shape and those who have a musculoskeletal problem may experience some problems with running, while others must be wary of its jarring effect on the feet, ankles, knees, and hips.

Food in Health and Disease

The body is an incredibly sensitive, complicated, and resilient machine. It is extremely adaptable to some factors in the environment, but just as susceptible to others. The most important weapon you have in the prevention of disease is your diet. As an athlete, you must understand the relationship between your food and nutrient intake and your health status.

As a population, Americans have an inordinately high rate of such illnesses as heart disease and cancer. This is due, in large part, to nutrient deficiencies and an overexposure to sugar, animal fat, and chemicals in our diet. Clearly, then, we must remove foods that contain chemicals, preservatives, and additives. One good way to begin is by eating organically grown vegetables, which are rich in fiber, easily digestible, and packed with vitamins and minerals. The vegetables can be eaten raw, steamed, sauteed, or as a juice.

Beyond that, carbohydrates should comprise about 70 percent of our diet. Excellent sources include legumes, beans, peas, lentils, broccoli, cabbage, cauliflower, turnips, watercress, rutabaga, sprouts, endive, escarole, radicchio, arugola, artichoke, seeds and nuts, and such grains as millet, kasha, oat, and wild rice.

Simple carbohydrates, on the other hand, should be removed from the diet. Overexposure to refined sugars (breads, cakes, and sweets) and even to a lot of fruit can increase blood sugar levels and prompt an oversecretion of insulin. In fact, many people have hypoglycemic episodes when extreme amounts of insulin are released. And too much insulin, in turn, can set the stage for the formation of plaque and the development of hypertension and heart disease. By removing all sugar from the diet, you can reduce weight and decrease your blood pressure, cholesterol, triglycerides, insulin overreaction, and, obviously, blood sugar levels.

Fats and oils, for their part, have gained a bad reputation in recent years that is only partially deserved. We do need some fats and oils in our bodies, even though these nutrients contain more calories than do proteins and carbohydrates. The best approach is to limit fats to about 15 percent of the calories in your diet and to derive this percentage from vegetable sources, such as safflower, sunflower, olive, and canola oils. The fats, oils, and meats from animals have been linked to various diseases, including colon polyps, cancer, breast cancer, and heart disease. They also greatly increase the tissue damage caused by free radicals.

The best sources of protein are beans, rice, peas, soy, nuts, and the like. Fish is another good source, but you need to be selective in deciding what types of fish to eat. Due to inland water contamination, deeper-sea fish are a safer—not to mention tastier—choice.

Finally, remember that stimulants such as caffeine can be a true diet disaster, whether they come from coffee, tea, or soda. Caffeine may cause dysinsulinism, palpitations, headaches, gut irritation, and nutrient malabsorption. It provides an artificial high that can become addicting. In addition to caffeine, soda contains large amounts of sugar and other undesirable substances that can affect your health. In lieu of these beverages, drink distilled water, seltzers, and fresh juice. Likewise, it's best to minimize unnecessary prescription medications because they can cause vitamin and mineral deficiencies.

As you pick up the pace with your exercise regimen, your caloric requirements may increase as well. With heavy endurance programs, some people go up to 3,000 or 4,000 calories. Solid foods should be consumed four hours before exercising, while liquids, such as distilled water or drinks with electrolytes or minerals, can be consumed two hours before exercising and during the workout. If you engage in a lengthy exercise routine that involves a lot of sweating, be sure to drink small cups of water throughout. Some experts recommend four to ten ounces of water every fifteen minutes of exercise and afterwards.

Nutrients for Exercise

When evaluating your nutrient status, the first course of action is to identify any vitamin or mineral deficiencies. That means measuring the body's levels of nutrients such as Vitamins A, C, and E, beta carotene, the B-Complex vitamins, and such minerals as selenium, manganese, zinc, boron, copper, calcium, and potassium.

A deficiency must be corrected by adjusting the foods in your diet and using specific oral, intramuscular, and intravenous treatments. The treatment needed will depend on the type of deficiency and whether malabsorption exists. Essentially, malabsorption is a diminished ability to take substances from the gut into the blood and tissues. In these cases, people who eat the right foods and take nutrients orally still may have deficiencies because their bodies are not absorbing the nutrients properly. This disorder is surprisingly common, in fact, and it requires the use of intramuscular and intravenous treatments that can bypass the digestive system.

As a result, people who exercise regularly—and those who are interested in preventive health—should assess their nutrient status. The traditional recommendations for nutritional requirements, such as the RDA, only allow for the dosages needed to prevent deficiency diseases, such as scurvy and beriberi. They do not provide guidelines for people who exercise or for the therapeutic benefits of nutrients.

Again, the correct level of nutrients will vary from one person to the next. Therefore, it is extremely important to be nutrient specific and to work with a physician when taking vitamins and minerals. Otherwise, the nutrients you take may be worthless, ineffective, or even harmful. With that said, however, all athletes and people who plan to begin exercising should consider their need for the following nutrients:

► Calcium, magnesium, and potassium: These are utilized during exercise and lost through sweating: 500 to 1,000 mg. for calcium; 200 to 500 mg. for magnesium; and 99 mg. for potassium.

► Germanium: can increase tissue oxygenation; 100 mg.

► DMG: can help to increase oxygenation of tissues.

► Chromium: stabilizes blood sugar levels and helps to metabolize fat; 200 mcg.

► Co-Q10: increases tissue oxygenation and improves cardiovascular function; 50 to 100 mg.

► L-Arginine and L-Ornithine: These amino acids can help to build muscle tissue and burn fat; 500 to 1,000 mg. each.

► L-Carnitine: helps bring fat to the muscle for use as energy; 500 to 1,000 mg.

- ► Amino acid mixtures: an easy way to absorb good protein sources.

- ► Betaine HCL and digestive enzymes: can increase the breakdown, digestion, and absorption of food.

- ► Zinc: promotes tissue growth and repair; 50 mg.

- ► Iron and folic acid: for hemoglobin and red-cell production; 800 to 1,000 mcg. of folic acid.

- ► Kelp: rich in iron for red-blood cell production and thyroid function; 150 mg.

In addition, B-Complex vitamins are important in combating stress, and such antioxidants as Vitamins A, C, E, and beta carotene are needed to bind to free radicals and prevent damage to healthy tissues. Indeed, the more intensely you work out, the more you need antioxidants because exercise generates free radical activity. Free radicals cause lipid peroxidation of cells and contribute to cell aging, atherosclerosis, and many other diseases.

Patient Experiences

In the end, what effect can nutrient deficiencies and diet have on your overall health and ability to perform as an athlete? Consider these five examples:

► Joe, a thirty-eight-year-old marathon runner training for his next race, had been suffering from chronic fatigue for five months when he sought professional help. Previously, Joe was in great condition. His illness started with what he described as a flu syndrome, accompanied by muscle aches, sinus congestion, chills, and a sore throat.

One doctor had already treated Joe with antibiotics and a cough medicine, neither of which provided any relief. The antibiotic, in fact, had given him an upset stomach and diarrhea. Joe ate the typical Westernized diet, consisting of meat, potatoes, and soda, but with little emphasis on vitamins and minerals. It's surprising that he was able to run or function well at all with such a diet.

Blood tests revealed that Joe had high cholesterol, high triglycerides, and low protein levels. Blood tests for vitamin and mineral levels showed that he had low levels of Vitamins C, B_6, and zinc. His physical exam was essentially negative, as were his blood pressure, temperature, stool tests, and urinalysis. And viral studies revealed positive results for cytomegalovirus and Epstein-Barr virus. Finally, food allergy testing showed that he was allergic to corn and milk.

What Joe needed was a drastic change in eating habits, and he was advised to remove corn, milk, red meat, preservatives, sugar, alcohol, and caffeine from his diet. He also began a vitamin protocol, including intravenous therapy. He got large doses of Vitamin C to stimulate immune function, inhibit the viruses, and generate a lot of antioxidant or free radical binding. Joe was also put on oral nutrients including B-Complex, digestive enzymes, and amino acids. The latter were used to increase protein absorption.

After his second week of intravenous therapy, Joe's energy levels started to improve, and he was able to resume running. His cholesterol and triglyceride levels were normalized by the sixth week. Joe maintained his new diet regimen as he continued to train, and he was able to surpass his previous training distance by seven miles.

▶ Susan, a twenty-nine-year-old teacher, suffered from migraine headaches for three months and was experiencing pain in her knees and wrists. She also had a history of eczema as a teenager. Susan was an avid runner, but she had stopped her routine schedule because of the headaches and joint pain. Lab testing revealed that Susan was anemic and had low cholesterol. She tested positive for allergies to tomatoes, wheat and soy, while vitamin and mineral testing showed that she was low in magnesium and had a B_{12} deficiency.

To correct these problems, Susan removed the offending foods from her diet, and her headaches were resolved after two weeks. She also received intramuscular injections of magnesium and B_{12}, which gave her an energy boost as well. While maintaining a vegetarian diet and taking oral nutrients, Susan resumed running and was able to enter the New York and Long Island marathons.

► Janet, a thirty-nine-year-old artist, had been gaining weight for a year. She was also losing hair and experiencing fatigue. Janet belonged to a race-walking group but was unable to keep up with her program. Routine testing revealed low thyroid function, elevated blood pressure, and high triglycerides.

Janet was placed on a no-sugar diet, a low-dose thyroid medication, and intravenous vitamins. Within two weeks, she felt an improvement in her energy level; within one month, her triglycerides were normal. She had stopped losing hair three weeks into the program.

► Adele is a fifty-nine-year-old woman who had been overweight for about twelve years. She had not been able to exercise for about five to seven years and was beginning to experience chest pain and shortness of breath when she exerted herself, such as when walking up stairs. A cardiologist had recommended that Adele receive bypass surgery for blockage in the coronary vessels. Adele was afraid of surgery (rightly so) and wanted to try a more nutritional approach to treatment. Testing showed that her cholesterol was 300, triglycerides were 270, and blood sugar ranged from 130 to 170. Adele's blood pressure was 170/110. The tests were repeated several times over three months to evaluate any changes, but all produced the same results. In addition, Adele's diet was atrocious. She ate red meat three times per week and cake and candy four times a week. She had few vegetables in her diet and never took vitamins.

The immediate response was to put her on a no-sugar diet, which allows the body to burn fat, including cholesterol and triglycerides. All animal meats and oils were removed from her diet, as were caffeine, preservatives, and junk food. She was told to drink vegetable juice at least twice a day, using carrots, red cabbage, celery, parsley, and others on a rotational basis.

The next step was to begin chelation therapy, following a twenty-four-hour urine test that showed her kidney function was normal. She received the chelation therapy twice each week. In the second week of treatment, her blood pressure went down to 150/90. It continued to normalize and reached 140/70 in the fourth week. Adele also lost thirty-seven pounds in approximately six weeks. She was free of chest pain and shortness of breath by the third week of treatment.

At the six-week mark, Adele began a slow and gradual walking program. Her chemistry was monitored routinely, and by the fifth week her cholesterol was down to 170 and triglyceride level was down to 100. Today, she walks ten to fifteen miles each day and also plays tennis and golf.

► Steve, a cyclist who worked for the parks department, suffered since childhood from sinus congestion and an allergy to mold and pollen. When tested for food and inhalant allergies, he tested positive for grass and weed pollens, milk, egg, and soy. His chemistry results were normal, but Steve was found to have low levels of Vitamin C, selenium, and zinc. As part of his treatment, Steve was desensitized weekly to the pollens. As a result, his sinus congestion and allergic symptoms cleared within two months. In addition, Steve was put on a vegetarian diet with vitamin supplements to correct his deficiencies and prevent disease. He is now a fierce competitor in his event.

So what have we learned? That optimum nutrition is a must for the excessive wear and tear on your muscles and bones and immune systems, that you must compensate for any extented or strenuous training.

1.   Eat to rehabilitate your immune system.

2.   Take proper amounts of the antioxidants. Get help from a qualified nutritionist, preferably a sports nutritionist.

3.   Treat your body with love and care. Don't train through injuries.

4.   Vegetarian diets with extra Vitamin B_{12}, iron, and proteins are excellent.

5.   Use guided visualization, meditation, yoga, and any good relaxation exercise to enhance inner harmony and self-esteem.

6.   Remember to play. Fun time is an excellent part of all training and living.

Appendix A

▼

How to Make the Natural Healing Oil

Ingredients

1 ounce tea tree oil
1 pint cold-pressed organic canola oil
½ ounce Pau D'Arco
½ ounce goldenseal root
50 Vitamin A capsules, 25,000 IU (all natural sources)
50 Vitamin D capsules, 5,000 IU (all natural sources)
50 Vitamin E capsules, 1,000 IU (d-alpha tocopherol)
cheesecloth
1-ounce ointment jar (from a pharmacy)
1-quart storage jar
4 ounces aloe vera gel

Directions

Heat the oil at a very low temperature (200 F. to 250 F.) for 10 to 20 hours with the Pau D'Arco and goldenseal root.

Boil the cheesecloth in water for 5 minutes, then allow it and the storage jar to cool.

Pour the oil and herbs into the cheesecloth slowly and strain the oil of all herbs as much as possible (two to four strainings) into the storage jar.

To the strained oil, add the Vitamins A, D, E, the tea tree oil, and the aloe gel.

Keep refrigerated.

211

Pour a small amount into the ointment jar and keep this at room temperature for daily use.

Discard the unused oil from the ointment jar each week.

Appendix B

▼

How to Make the Herbal Soak for Fungus Nails

Ingredients
___

Pau D'Arco (2 to 3 tea bags)
Peppermint (1 tea bag)
Goldenseal root (1 tea bag)
Comfrey leaves (1 tea bag)
Tea tree oil

Directions
___

Add all tea bags to 3 cups of boiling water. Allow to cool until solution is warm. Soak teas for 30 minutes, twice a day.

After soaking, paint cuticle with tea tree oil (like nail polish, except around the nail, not on it).

Appendix C

Logbook Work Sheet

Date _____

Time of day _____

Pulse rate before running _____

Pulse rate after running at   6 minutes _____

                                     8 minutes _____

                                  10 minutes _____

Energy level $+1$, $+2$, $+3$, $+4$, $+5$ _____

Terrain _____

Weather conditions _____

Distance run _____

Time _____

Miles a minute _____

Speed work (include time and distances) _____

Interval training _____

Total miles run in shoes _____

Comments (including thoughts, feelings, and ideas, discomforts,

pains, etc.) _____

_____

_____

Index

218

Kargere, Dr. Audrey, 78
Katch, Frank J., 176
Kelp, 207
Kendall, Dr. Roger, 174, 175, 176,
   178, 179, 180, 181, 182
Kidney and hyperthermia, 47, 83
Kinesiology, 27, 77
Knees, holistic warm-up of, 58
Kraus, Dr. Hans, 22–23
Krishnamurti, *xiii, xvi*

Lactose and diarrhea, 45
Legs
   holistic warm-up of, 60
   post-run stretches of, 63–64
Legumes
   as complex carbohydrates, 134
   as fiber, 197
Ligaments
   general prevention of injury,
      23–24
   injury to, 21–23
Lipoproteins (high & low-density)
   and blood work-up, 42
Liquids
   alcoholic & caffeinated, 51
   chills & chapping, 53
   cold versus hot, 50
   and exercise, 12, 15, 47, 48,
      49, 83
   and kidney functioning, 83
   and marathon running, 92
   post-exercise, 85
   with sugar content, 50–51
   and weather, 120
Logbook, 66, 90
Logbook Work Sheet, 214
Lysine, 181–82

McArdle, William K., 13, 176
McBride, Dr. Angus, Jr., 29
McNeil, Dr., 175–76
Magnesium, 15, 50, 84, 166, 206
   as supplement, 120, 121, 175,
      208
   and weight management,
      11–16
Magnetism therapy, 29, 80
Male runners
   and athletic supporters, 37

and calcium, 8
and hormonal changes, 46
as interval training
Manganese, 166–67
   as supplement, 120
Marathon running
   as aerobic alternative, 106–07
   diet, 94
   form, 92–93
   pacing, 90–92
   training, 88–90
   See also Exercise program;
      Running; Stretching; Training
Massage, 80–81
Medical treatment
   attention to injury, 12, 20
   cardiac physical, 42
   cortisone injections, 30
   environmental, 188–89
   orthopedics, 28–29
   orthotic devices, 26, 27, 29, 32
   patient experiences, 207–10
   See also Diagnosis; Healers;
      Injury; Therapies; Surgery
Meditation, 4, 55–56, 77–78, 210
Menopause and calcium, 8
Menstrual irregularities, 36–37, 46
Metartarsals, holistic warm-up of, 59
Metatarsus adductus, 25–26
Moisturizer and chapping, 53
Muscle endurance training, 102
Muscles
   composition of, 13–14
   cramps, 15–16
   DOMS, 16
   general prevention of injury,
      23–24
   hamstring injury, 18–19
   plantar fasciitis, 17–18
   shin splints, 16–17
   strains, 15
   tight rear leg, 26
Musculoskeletal system and
   running, 7

National Association for Sports and
   Physical Education, 173
Natural Healing Oil, 211–12
Natural Living Running and Walking
   Club, 121

Sodium, 50, 169
Spine, problems of, 28–29, 55
Sports medicine. *See* Medical
treatment
Sprinting, 98
Strength endurance training, 102
Stress (emotional) and running, 7,
8, 10, 177
Stress fractures and women, 29
Stretching, 12
and hamstring injury, 18
hurdler's stretch, 22
and lower back, 28, 55
passive, 59
post-exercise, 23–24, 63–66
and spasms, 30
and tendinitis, 20
See also Exercise program;
Running; Training
Sugar
avoidance of, 31, 32, 116, 121,
132, 189–90, 191–92
and blood work-up, 42
and criminality, 191–92
and health, 191–92, 209
types of, 190
when necessary, 75
Sulfur and hyperthermia, 50
Sunburn, 33
Supplements (nutritional), 120–21,
172–84, 197–98
Swimming, 28, 101, 104–05, 203

Temporomandibular joint
imbalance, 27
Tendinitis
general prevention, 23–24
treatment of, 19–21
Tension, relief of, 4
Terrain and exercise, 11, 22, 32
Therapies
acupuncture, 17, 77
Alexander Technique, 28, 77
applied kinesiology, 27, 77
autogenic training, 77–78
biofeedback training, 78
brain synchronizer, 78
chelation therapy, 209
color therapy, 78
cranial therapy, 78

diathermy, 78–79
electrical muscle stimulation,
79
galvanic electric therapy, 79
heat therapy, 79
homeopathy, 79
hydrotherapy, 79
hypnotherapy, 79–80
ice therapy, 80
magnetism, 80
massage, 80–81
patient experiences, 207–10
physical therapy, 81
polarity therapy, 81
ultrasound therapy, 42, 81
Townsend Letter for Doctors, 181
Toxins, removal from body, 7
Training
after injury, 24
and attitude, 4
detraining & overtraining,
43–44
and scheduling, 4
and a sense of play, 210
See also Exercise program;
Marathon running;
Stretching; Running
Training, forms of
aerobic, 8, 10, 45, 97–98,
100–01
circuit training, 102
Fartlek method,101
interval training, 101
local muscle endurance, 102
strength endurance, 102
Transformation process
as buzzword, *xiv*
and non-integrated belief
systems, *xv*
and running, *xvi*
True self
and ego, *xv*
evaluation of, 3–4
Tryglycerides, 42, 171
24-hour halter monitor, 42
28-day plan for runners, 66–70
option A, 70–71
option B, 72–73

Ultrasound therapy, 42, 81

CHAPTER 13

'I'iwi: (ee-ee-vee) A native Hawaiian bird with bright vermillion feathers still fairly common on Kauai, Maui, and the Big Island. Feathers were used extensively by ancient Hawaiians in making their capes and helmets.

CHAPTER 17

Mahalo: (mah-HAW-loe) Hawaiian for thanks.

Pidgin English: (PID-juhn) A simplified version of English. It was originally used in the Orient for communication between people who spoke different languages.

Breakaway

With colorful graphics, hot topics and humor, this magazine for teen guys helps them keep their faith on course *and* gives the latest info on sports, music, celebrities . . . even girls. Best of all, this publication shows teens how they can put their Christian faith into practice and resist peer pressure.

Clubhouse

Here's a fun way to instill Christian principles in your children! With puzzles, easy-to-read stories and exciting activities, *Clubhouse* provides hours of character-building enjoyment for kids ages 8 to 12.

All magazines are published monthly except where otherwise noted. For more information regarding these and other resources, please call Focus on the Family at (719) 531-5181, or write to us at Focus on the Family, Colorado Springs, CO 80995.